FIBRE FOR LIFE

DR. KHOSRO EZAZ-NIKPAY

LIVE LONGER AND HEALTHIER WITH NATURE'S MIRACLE INGREDIENT

PAVILION

First published in the United Kingdom in 2021 by
Pavilion
43 Great Ormond Street
London
WC1N 3HZ

ISBN 978-1-911663-56-0

A CIP catalogue record for this book is available from the
British Library.
10 9 8 7 6 5 4 3 2 1

Reproduction by Rival Colour Ltd., London
Printed and bound by Toppan Leefung Printing Ltd., China
www.pavilionbooks.com

Illustrator: Andrew Baker
Publisher: Helen Lewis
Commissioning editor: Sophie Allen
Design manager: Laura Russell
Cover design: Luke Bird
Production manager: Phil Brown

DISCLAIMER: The information in this book is
provided as an information resource only and is
not to be used or relied on for any diagnostic,
treatment or medical purpose. All health issues
should be discussed with your GP and/or other
qualified medical professional.

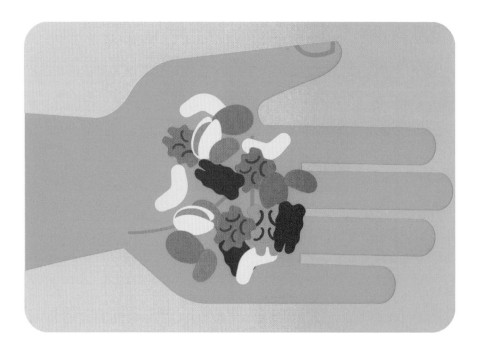

CONTENTS

7 KEY POINTS ABOUT FIBRE

1. We over-eat most macronutrients: sugar, protein and fat. We are badly deficient in fibre.

2. This is shortening our lives by many years.

3. Current strategies that focus on reducing overconsumption have proven futile:

+ diets don't work over the long-term because they expect a change in habits and lifestyle.
+ a sugar tax has not reduced obesity because there are many ways to circumvent the tax.
+ sweeteners and supplements are not the solution because our metabolism can outsmart them.
+ preaching and shaming has not worked because – when has it ever worked?

4. There is a simple strategy that is certain to work because it already does: increasing our fibre consumption:

+ people who eat more fibre live longer and healthier by a huge margin (for every 10g of additional fibre you reduce mortality by 10%, which is over 7 years of healthy life).

+ over the past few years, science has started to explain why fibre is so central to our lives and every day we uncover new wonders.

+ by physically changing our gut and feeding our gut bacteria, fibre has a profound impact on our entire system (metabolism, immune, digestive, nervous and cardiovascular systems).

+ our gut bacteria act as a quasi organ. The main food this organ needs is fibre and it is starving (let me repeat starving!) in most of us.

5. This strategy is affordable at the individual and societal level and would save our economies billions, but more importantly prolong our lives by powerfully tackling most of the big diseases that haunt us.

6. With three simple strategies, this book will help to add up to 10 healthy years to your life:

I. **Fibre up** – easy ways of adding fibre to your diet and some recipes.

II. **Physical activity up** – ways to sneak in more activity into your day, no sweat.

III. **Fun up** – easy ways to motivate yourself and improve your sleep.

7. In summary, there is no drug as powerful as fibre and this book will give you all the evidence and tools you need to add it to your life without having to change your lifestyle or habits dramatically.

'WHAT IS SEVEN EXTRA YEARS OF HEALTHY LIFE WORTH TO YOU?'

As a child, I discovered that, when playing hide-and-seek, one of the best strategies was to hide in plain sight. It was an eerie experience; how was it that the friend looking for me in the playground couldn't spot me? I can only guess that when we are too focused on finding the hidden, we often miss the obvious. This book is about how one of our greatest nutritional treasures is doing exactly the same thing: hiding in plain sight.

What am I talking about? Fibre. That's right – boring, tasteless, invisible fibre. And yet exciting new research has found that, while we've had our eye caught by endless fad diets and supplements with empty promises, it's actually fibre that can help us live longer and, most importantly, ensure those years are healthy ones.

It does this by improving the health of our heart and blood circulation, reducing inflammation and strengthening our hormonal and immune systems. By doing so, it can save tens of billions in our healthcare systems and, more importantly, save many, many lives.

On top of all of that, fibre is an affordable and powerful tool for improving a society's health. Forget about cutting out this or restricting that, adding fibre to our diets is easier and better for us than trying to reduce fat, sugar or carbs.

This book will hopefully convince you that taking a closer look at fibre may be one of the best things you can do for your health and, indirectly, the health of our planet, too.

THE JOURNEY TO FIBRE

My mother, like many others, smoked. Even though at that time it was not yet fully understood how dangerous it could be, I knew it wasn't good. I started tinkering with various inventions to filter out as much smoke as possible and badgered her to smoke through them, which she complied with until I went to bed.

Even at such a young age, I was fascinated by two seemingly contradictory facts: firstly, with so many people getting sick from smoking, why did they not just stop (or use my complicated contraptions)? And secondly, why did it take years before diseases manifested themselves? Why did some people live to an old age before they got sick?

As none of my teachers could provide satisfying answers to these questions it was clear to me that, if I really wanted to understand this, I would have to dig deeper.

THE KEY TO HEALTH

I decided to study chemistry at the University of California, Berkeley, where complex chemical processes were brought vividly to life by the wondrous world of our biology.

In my last semester of undergraduate studies there was a fire in my laboratory and I was badly burnt. If this had happened before the advent of antibiotics, you would not be reading this book. During my time in hospital, I became fascinated by how my body healed itself. Skin cells around hair roots that were spared began growing like crazy to fill the damaged spaces between them; a high fever indicated a fight with bacteria trying to invade the breached barrier of my skin; and a ravishing hunger gave me the energy to repair myself. When I arrived at my graduate school at Harvard University, six months later, I was determined to further delve into how cells function and repair damage.

My doctoral thesis focused on this and I found our cells have a whole armament of repair functions to protect us with. Proteins patrol our DNA to detect and repel any attack or error. As I worked on my PhD it started to answer some of my childhood questions: the reason we do not get immediately sick when abusing our bodies is because there are multiple lines of defence at the cellular and immune system level. Only when these are overwhelmed can disease take a foothold. The key to healthy longevity is keeping those systems working at their optimum level.

SCIENCE AND THE REAL WORLD

After graduating, I decided to switch track to better understand what it takes to translate pure scientific knowledge into the messy world of society, politics and economics. I joined McKinsey & Company, a management consultancy, and worked on the broadest set of economic problems imaginable. In many ways, I discovered that the very same powerful mechanisms I encountered in my studies had equivalent themes in business: the evolution of species and the dynamics of markets; ecosystems in nature and ecosystems in industry sectors; the immune system and risk management – they were essentially the same. It was exhilarating to see these parallels and how one can inspire the other. I also learnt that, outside of a crisis, it is easiest to change companies if the change can be incorporated into the fabric and existing habits of the company and its staff. This simple insight will be highly relevant when we discuss why it is better to increase fibre intake rather than try to lower sugar intake or engage in a diet that requires a change in lifestyle.

When I left McKinsey to start my own companies, it was a scary prospect. I started from zero, armed with a single question: what are the main drivers of human health and is it possible to create products that powerfully support them? As my team and I started to research this in-depth, we realised that, while there is a wealth of knowledge on the function of cells and organisms, there is very little reliable information at population level. You can find a huge body of excellent science on this or that 'super'-ingredient reducing the incidence of this or that disease, but there is very little on if there are also adverse effects. For example, while aspirin reduces the incidence of cardiovascular disease (and headaches), does its propensity to cause bleeding undo some or all of the benefits?

It became increasingly clear that one must look at the big picture and determine benefit against parameters that are rarely measured. How many years of healthy life are added through an intervention? Is there a positive impact on all-cause mortality? Is the intervention societally affordable or only for the few?

THE F-WORD

How does all this relate to fibre? Well, during our research, my team and I found ourselves tripping over this nutrient again and again. The penny really only dropped when we connected the dots and could see the central role that fibre plays in our various bodily systems: from the gut and digestion to our cardiovascular, hormonal, immune and nervous systems.

Once we started to analyse its impact on healthy longevity and all-cause mortality, there was no escaping the life-changing insight that fibre is *the* nutrient which has the widest and most profound positive impact on our health. Fibre crowds out bad nutrition and shifts our food intake to the types of foods that are also better for the environment and health of the planet. Plus, the more fibre you consume, the better the outcome.

For all the products that my colleagues and I have created, no matter what the intended consumer benefit, we pay attention to the level of fibre, specifically the sugar-to-fibre ratio.

For example, we created the first commercial

vegan ice cream, Frill, which had ten times the fibre and less than half the sugar (which came from fresh fruit) of a typical ice cream. It was one of the lowest calorie products on the market without having to resort to using sweeteners, and while it was extremely low in sugar, what we really cared about was that it was very high in fibre. With every new bit of evidence that emerges about the health benefits of fibre, we are increasingly proud of our tasty creation, where a single portion delivers about a third of your daily fibre needs. But there are many ways of upping your fibre intake and the important thing is not our creation, but that you find a way to eat more fibre. I will tell you why and give you many ideas of how.

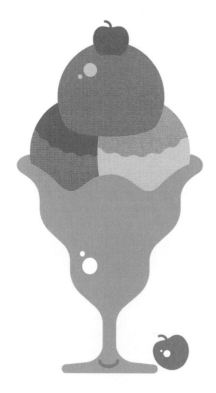

WHAT'S IN A WORD?

The word *fibre* as the British write it, or *fiber* as the North Americans write it, originates from the Latin *fibre* or *fibra*. This meant filament or entrails, which was also the older proto-Indo-European meaning of tendon, sinew and bowstring, presumably because they were often made from the intestines of animals.

Fibre is also what the gut – our intestines – needs to be healthy. In this sense, fibre is descriptive and prescriptive; it's what they are and also what they need to survive. Our new scientific understanding has brought fibre full circle back to its roots.

MY SALES PITCH

Put simply, fibre is difficult to patent and sell at a premium the way a new drug might be. It's also not particularly tasty, unlike sugar or fat. Plus, in the short term its impact is subtle; its profundity is only revealed in the mid to long term.

I'm passionate about persuading you to up your intake of fibre. If fibre were to be marketed as a new pharmaceutical product, the response to it would be akin to that of a miracle drug, so profound are its effects on our health, well-being and longevity.

Fibre makes you feel fuller faster. It promotes satiety which, in turn, helps you maintain a healthy weight; this on its own promotes a whole range of health benefits.

But that's just the beginning: fibre feeds your gut bacteria, the body's own internal doctors, which in turn deliver a wide range of benefits to your cardiovascular, immune, digestive, metabolic, and (potentially) nervous, systems. The links between higher fibre consumption and significantly reduced risk of numerous debilitating diseases are many, and every day new ones are being discovered. Our gut bacteria, for example, protect our digestive system from less friendly pathogens. By interacting with our various body systems via the different chemicals they produce (such as short-chain fatty acids that play an important role in modulating inflammation), they help to significantly reduce the risk of some of the biggest human killers. These include cardiovascular disease (heart attacks, strokes) and some cancers (colorectal, breast and lung)[1]. So, when I talk about the various health benefits of fibre, it is shorthand for how the various fibres feed our many beneficial gut bacteria, which in turn keep us healthy.

For something that we've all heard of, many know very little about it. Where do I find it? How much is enough? Is it the same as roughage? Doesn't it give me wind?

Over the following pages you'll learn about the incredible benefits of fibre, where to get your hands on it and how you can make it work for you. Most importantly, this book will give you the practical tools and tips to start making the easy changes you need, today. There are recipes, shopping lists, easy snack swaps and nifty tricks for sneaking more fibre into your everyday food intake. In short, I hope it will help you become as interested in fibre as I am, keen to tell the world about its benefits and skilled in transforming your own diet and health without having to change your lifestyle, likes and dislikes.

To circle back to my childhood questions, why did my mother not use my anti-smoke contraption? Because she would have had to change her habits and look ridiculous in front of other smokers. When habits clash with health, habits often win, so we have to find ways to improve our health that work with habits and lifestyles.

And why are we so resilient in the face of disease? Because our bodies have many layers of defence systems and these create a false sense of security. While one scoop of ice cream will certainly make very little difference to your long-term health, constant bad nutritional choices and lack of exercise and sleep will build up enough pressure to burst your invincibility bubble. On the other hand, doing a few simple things right will help your innate defences to do their job like a charm.

One of those simple things is increasing your intake of fibre. This book is a homage to that, and an urgent attempt to stop people looking for the hidden and to refocus on the obvious.

THE IMPORTANCE OF THE SUGAR-TO-FIBRE RATIO

The sugar-to-fibre ratio is a term you'll hear a lot as you read this book. And you'll soon come to realise, it's the most important thing to bear in mind when it comes to your food choices.

Much of the world's attention is on reducing sugar and, while this is a noble cause as a way of tackling obesity, it will, in my opinion, ultimately end in failure. Pretty much all the diets that we have plagued ourselves with, since the advent of obesity and various cultural beauty diktats, require people to change their lifestyle or habits. This is something an individual might be able to achieve here and there, but at a societal level all evidence points to a different conclusion. I hope to convince you that it is not the amount of sugar (or fat, or calories or whatever is the latest diet-industry obsession), but the ratio of sugar-to-fibre that is important.

I believe adding fibre is a more powerful strategy than removing sugar, and I'll return to this throughout the book. Even with plant materials, the sugar-to-fibre ratio – that is to say, how much fibre bang you get for your sugar buck – can make a big difference when it comes to foods being healthy or less so. Vegetables and fruit that have sugar in them are healthy because that sugar comes with fibre.

A NOTE ABOUT META-ANALYSIS

In making the claims in this book I rely primarily on meta-analysis and using multiple lines of evidence. What this means is that, as a scientist, I do not trust a lone scientific study. The result may be due to luck or inadequate methods and controls. Recent analysis shows that a significant portion of scientific work cannot be easily replicated[2]. Also people generally do not publish negative results. It is therefore more prudent to look at the entire body of evidence, try to find any evidence that contradicts the findings and look at what is called 'dose-response' relationships. Dose-response simply means that if I do more of a good thing, I should see more of a positive effect. Therefore, if I don't see this, there may not be a relationship between doing what I think is beneficial and the desired effect. For example, there are many meta-analyses and dose-response relationships supporting my claim regarding the benefits of fibre on cardiovascular health, whereas the evidence for the benefit of fibre on attention deficit hyperactivity disorder (ADHD) is more tenuous; therefore I have mentioned it with far more caution.

As more and more evidence gathers around the benefits of fibre, I will publish the latest review of major investigations at www.fiber4life.com/fiber-facts so that you have the latest evidence at your fingertips.

1. HIDING IN PLAIN SIGHT

'WHEN YOU ARE TOO FOCUSED ON FINDING THE HIDDEN, YOU OFTEN MISS THE OBVIOUS.'

F ibre. It doesn't sound very exciting, does it? And yet if you want to live a long and healthy life it should become music to your ears. Simply put, increasing your fibre intake will benefit gut health and strengthen immunity, thus helping with conditions such as obesity, diabetes, heart disease and inflammation. Not only that, moving to a more plant-based diet (high in fibre) can positively affect societal and environmental concerns too. Let's talk about why...

The single most important determinant in your ability to live a long – and, more importantly, healthy – life is the food you choose to eat. My goal with this book is to persuade you that fibre, this undervalued nutrient, deserves the most prominent place in your diet. Let's prioritise fibre – put it on a pedestal – because, as you'll learn, the benefits are too good to be missing out on.

It seems to me that fibre has fallen out of favour. Why? Well, as we'll discuss throughout this book, there are myriad reasons, ranging from perception problems to changing tastes. But a common thread is that, as fibre has been sidelined from our diets, so too has our knowledge of why it's so wonderful. We've become unaccustomed to consuming it as more convenient options have become available, so we've forgotten how good it makes us feel.

Historically, we humans used to consume far more fibre than we do today. If you look at traditional diets in most regions of the world, people ate a high-fibre diet because they tended to eat the whole grain and vegetables straight from the field, and fruit straight from the tree. Sugar, meat or processed foods were either unavailable or inaccessible for most of our ancestors.

WHERE FIBRE IS FOUND: EXAMPLE USING THE CORN PLANT

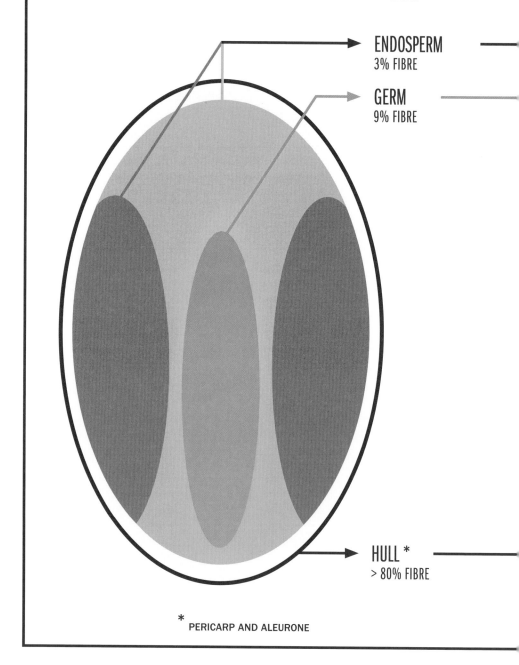

ENDOSPERM
3% FIBRE

GERM
9% FIBRE

HULL *
> 80% FIBRE

* PERICARP AND ALEURONE

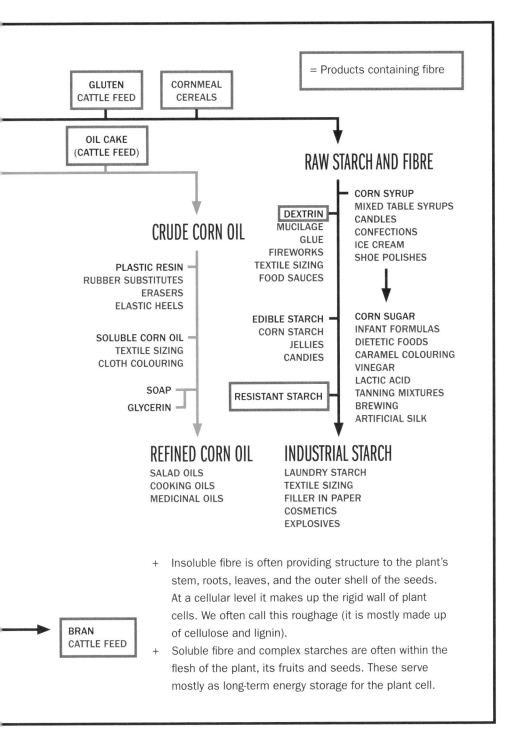

GLUTEN
CATTLE FEED

CORNMEAL
CEREALS

= Products containing fibre

OIL CAKE
(CATTLE FEED)

RAW STARCH AND FIBRE

CORN SYRUP
MIXED TABLE SYRUPS
CANDLES
CONFECTIONS
ICE CREAM
SHOE POLISHES

DEXTRIN
MUCILAGE
GLUE
FIREWORKS
TEXTILE SIZING
FOOD SAUCES

CRUDE CORN OIL

PLASTIC RESIN
RUBBER SUBSTITUTES
ERASERS
ELASTIC HEELS

CORN SUGAR
INFANT FORMULAS
DIETETIC FOODS
CARAMEL COLOURING
VINEGAR
LACTIC ACID
TANNING MIXTURES
BREWING
ARTIFICIAL SILK

EDIBLE STARCH
CORN STARCH
JELLIES
CANDIES

SOLUBLE CORN OIL
TEXTILE SIZING
CLOTH COLOURING

SOAP
GLYCERIN

RESISTANT STARCH

REFINED CORN OIL

SALAD OILS
COOKING OILS
MEDICINAL OILS

INDUSTRIAL STARCH

LAUNDRY STARCH
TEXTILE SIZING
FILLER IN PAPER
COSMETICS
EXPLOSIVES

BRAN
CATTLE FEED

+ Insoluble fibre is often providing structure to the plant's stem, roots, leaves, and the outer shell of the seeds. At a cellular level it makes up the rigid wall of plant cells. We often call this roughage (it is mostly made up of cellulose and lignin).

+ Soluble fibre and complex starches are often within the flesh of the plant, its fruits and seeds. These serve mostly as long-term energy storage for the plant cell.

MORE PROCESSING, LESS FIBRE

As our food has become more refined and processed, what is inevitably lost is the fibre. A grain of wheat is full of fibre, but by the time the wheat germ has been removed and it's been processed into white flour, much of the fibre has been washed out. Of course, you now have a product that's easy to make into pasta, white bread, pizza bases and certain breakfast cereals – products that are tasty and easily digested – but in doing so you've lost the most important health element to the food: the fibre.

Our taste buds have been trained to recognise foods that we associate with being beneficial or rewarding to us. With sugar and fat there's a reaction that says, 'Oh, energy', and with protein/amino acids the response is, 'Oh, something with which I can repair my body'. The connections are positive ones and these form habits.

The tongue has no such detectors for fibre, so it stands to reason that food manufacturers are predisposed to focus on products that satisfy a need the body recognises. The downside of this is that fibre has less commercial potential than fat, sugar and protein, hence its scarcity in processed foods. Sure, it's a nutrient boon for our intestinal bacteria (more on this in Chapter 4), but it's not a nutrient for us in the way that protein, fat and carbohydrates are. The tongue rather than the gut has come to rule the body.

FIBRE AND MORTALITY

The most robust way to measure the benefits of any health intervention and ensure that it has an overall net positive benefit is to ask if all-cause mortality is reduced. (All-cause mortality includes every kind of death, from infectious diseases to accidents. It is the one number that is not subject to interpretation. All other statistics run the risk of miscounting the cause.) While most interventions and drugs fail this test, fibre excels: an extra 10g of fibre a day can reduce all-cause mortality by approximately 10%[3]. If every American ate a handful of raspberries every day, the health impact would be equivalent to saving the same number of lives that perish in traffic accidents over seven years[4].

In line with this, in 2019, the World Health Organization (WHO), based on a broad review of meta-analyses, stated that a diet rich in fibre results in a 15–30% reduction in early deaths, with rates of coronary heart disease, stroke, type 2 diabetes and colorectal cancer reduced by 16–24% (see [12]). Not bad, I think you'll agree?

So how does fibre do all this? I'll reveal more in later chapters, but some of the broad benefits are based on its anti-inflammatory actions, as mediated by the gut microbiota. Inflammation is a normal and desirable process. It's effectively your body's way of dealing with problems, such as a microorganism invading your body or cells rupturing after trauma.

Where inflammation becomes a problem is when the body is in a low-level inflammatory state all the time, without having sustained any trauma. Emerging evidence suggests this is linked to a whole host of chronic health conditions. And, importantly, fibre seems to significantly reduce an unwanted inflammatory response.

In this way, fibre can lead to massive reductions in diseases of the cardiovascular system, including reduced arterial plaque formation, cutting down the chances of a cardiac event.

And scientists are finding more and more evidence for the central health role of fibre. While some of the evidence is at a very early stage (such as its benefit for improving sleep, depression, anxiety or its positive impact on respiratory diseases, including lower risk of chronic obstructive pulmonary disease (COPD)[5], influenza and COVID-19)[6], I'm convinced that in thirty years' time, we will look back and wonder why this miracle drug wasn't given more attention.

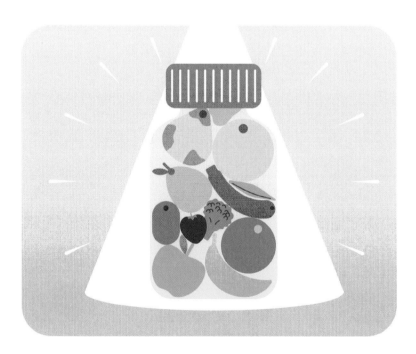

THE REAL SWEET STUFF

On a micro level, the positive relationship between fibre and disease risk alone is worth getting your fix. But let's step back and look at the bigger picture, too.

I see people enjoying significantly longer, healthier lives; able to contribute more to society and reduce the burden on the state. I see the potential global impact of fibre.

A fibre-rich (and more plant-based) diet not only benefits us as individuals, it's also an affordable option for most households and therefore a powerful tool for improving the health of society as a whole.

Even a mild shift to a more fibre-rich diet not only improves our health, but also naturally lowers our consumption of animal-based products and resulting environmental impact without taxing our purses.[7] The reason is that in terms of land, energy and water usage, fibre-containing foods reduce natural resource usage by close to 80% and greenhouse gas emissions by 50–95% for the same nutrient content when compared to animal-derived foods.[8]

WHY DO I CARE ABOUT THE SUGAR-TO-FIBRE RATIO

While there is much debate among scientists, nutritionists and policy makers as to which macronutrient culprit to focus on, the big picture is rather simple to understand.[9] In 1965, the average person living on earth consumed 2358 kcal/day, today, over half a century later, the average person consumes a quarter more.[10,11] Our over-consumption derives from three sources:

FAT. Fats and oils are energy dense (that is why we store them in our fat cells) and healthy. However, we are currently over-consuming fat by 80–130%. Over-consumption is not healthy and a broad body of research points to many potential deleterious effects, particularly on the cardiovascular system.[12]

SUGAR (AND SIMPLE CARBS). Sugar is an important nutrient and an easy source of energy. However, we are over-consuming sugar by over 80%. This has many negative effects particularly in promoting type 2

THE FIBRE RULE OF THUMB

Any ratio lower than 4:1 is healthy

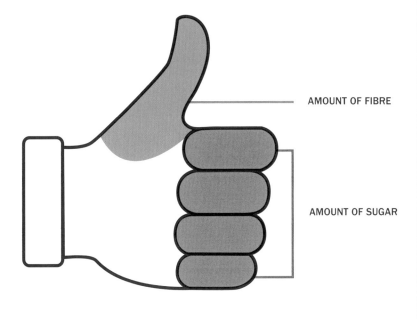

AMOUNT OF FIBRE

AMOUNT OF SUGAR

VEGETABLES **1:3**

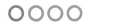

FRUIT **4:1**

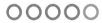

SNACKS **20:1**

diabetes and the connected impact on our cardiovascular system.[13]

PROTEIN. Protein is a critical nutrient that helps build tissue and sustain many physiological processes in the body. Especially in the fitness space, where protein is required for muscle build-up and damage repair. Non-athletes, however, are over-consuming protein by 50–100% with potential harmful impact, despite what the marketing people tell you.[14]

And we under-consume fibre by up to 50%. So as far as I am concerned, what we need to fix is the imbalance and not get lost in trying to focus on any one nutrient. The reason that I propose the sugar-to-fibre ratio is simple: fibre has proven powerful, life-prolonging benefits and sugar consumption probably is the best indicator of bad nutrition-behaviour irrespective of its direct role in our health.

There are many caveats to consider, of course, but these are minor compared to the big picture presented here. For example, despite the low overall all-cause mortality of the Japanese lifestyle over the past 60 years (see next segment), specifically, cerebrovascular mortality has dropped significantly, potentially linked to higher animal product consumption (dairy, meat and eggs). However, the Japanese still consume significantly lower amounts of animal protein (by about 45%) than a typical Western diet. In other words, they are not yet in over-consumption territory and as we will see, it is their high-fibre consumption that keeps them healthy.

THE WEALTH OF NATIONS

As surprising as this sounds, a quick comparison of the sugar-to-fibre ratios of developed nations bears this out: the more fibre a country eats compared to sugar, the higher its life expectancy and, more importantly, its healthy longevity. The Japanese have seven additional years of healthy longevity than the US (and 4.7 additional years than the Italians). That is seven additional years of life that can be enjoyed free from disease. The same correlation is seen, for example, in the occurrence of obesity. This can have huge ramifications for a nation's economy as well as its health. As we will see, the per capita spending on obesity increases in line with the sugar-to-fibre consumption of a country, meaning that, if allowed to, fibre can have a positive effect for society financially. We do not see a similar clear correlation when looking at other ratios of macronutrients.[15]

The worse (higher) the sugar-to-fibre ratio is in a country, the higher the rate of obesity.[16] That is a fact. And it costs money: per capita spending on obesity in the US – a country that has a 6:1 sugar-to-fibre ratio – is $1,335 (adjusted for factor costs – see page 33). That's a lot of money to treat a condition that is potentially avoidable. Not only is that a financial burden on a nation, but as we slowly emerge from a global pandemic, such a wilful drain on resources is selfish at best, and immoral at worst.

SUGAR-TO-FIBRE RATIO IS A GOOD PROXY FOR SOCIETAL HEALTH

 JAPAN   ITALY

USA

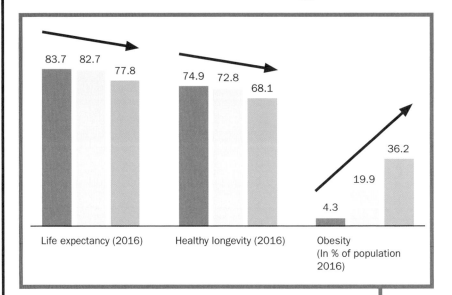

83.7	82.7	77.8
Life expectancy (2016)		

74.9	72.8	68.1
Healthy longevity (2016)		

4.3	19.9	36.2
Obesity (In % of population 2016)		

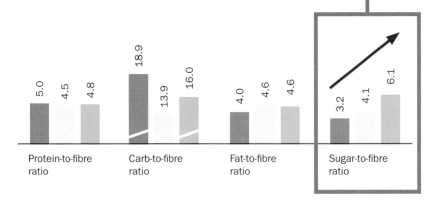

5.0	4.5	4.8
Protein-to-fibre ratio		

18.9	13.9	16.0
Carb-to-fibre ratio		

4.0	4.6	4.6
Fat-to-fibre ratio		

3.2	4.1	6.1
Sugar-to-fibre ratio		

Note: The numbers are based on added sugar. The total sugar consumed is less well known and is even higher, skewing the data further in favour of Japan.

THE SUGAR-TO-FIBRE RATIO HAS HUGE RAMIFICATIONS FOR OUR ECONOMIES

PER CAPITA SPENDING ON OBESITY ADJUSTED FOR FACTOR COSTS ($)

In order to compare the different healthcare systems in a fairer way, costs were adjusted to reflect inherent different costs (factor costs) for drugs, insurance, salaries etc. in order to reflect primarily the true costs of the disease.

1335

676

502

	Japan	Italy	USA
SUGAR-TO-FIBRE RATIO	**3.2**	**4.1**	**6.1**

Compare the US to Japan and Italy – 3:1 and 4:1 sugar-to-fibre ratios respectively – and that drops to $502 and $676 per capita. From a nutritional perspective, populations with higher longevity are not doing anything particularly revolutionary, save eating a lot of vegetables, pulses, nuts, seeds and grains. The rice and pasta that comprise their national dishes crowd out most of the bad food choices, while the nuts, seeds, pulses, grains, fruit and vegetables provide the fibre, keeping that sugar-to-fibre ratio on the right side of healthy (i.e., lower than 4). It's obviously working for them, but imagine the boost in their healthy longevity if they swapped their white pasta and white rice for brown varieties. Even the healthiest and happiest people in the world can reap the benefits of an increased fibre intake.

POVERTY AND LOWER FIBRE INTAKE

Interestingly, we can also draw parallels between income levels and cases of obesity, health and longevity. Referring to the data, Italy and Japan are much more similar in terms of size and economic equality. But the US is more polarised: in my experience, if you are in affluent downtown Los Angeles you will have a hard time finding an obese person, but if you go into the poorer parts of the Valley area, you'll struggle to find a thin one. It's a two-tier society and, in many ways, the UK is similar. I work near the Westway in west London's borough of Kensington and Chelsea and, for people living north of that area, life expectancy is ten years lower than for those living to the south in the affluent areas of Notting Hill.[17] That is the difference between North Korea and Luxembourg.

There's an unfortunate correlation: people who have a lower income tend to develop obesity-related diseases. They also eat less dietary fibre. Obviously, fibre deficiency is just one factor here – there are other correlations between lower income and reduced longevity which take into account factors such as stress and greater exposure to infectious diseases. But it's difficult not to see that a lack of fibre is an important element in the reduced healthy longevity of low-income households.[18] A large body of epidemiological data also demonstrates that diet quality is associated with greater affluence. Diets that are energy dense but nutrient poor are preferentially consumed by households with lower socio-economic status. The poorer you are, the higher the incentives to pay the minimum money for the maximum energy, which means high sugar/high fat – with all the negative ramifications.[19]

Once you look at things from a fibre perspective, namely the key nutrient you want to actually pay for, the picture changes. While it is certainly true that fresh fruit costs more per calorie than cheap sugar and fat, unrefined products are, on the whole, no more expensive than their refined brethren (see Chapter 5).

It seems our palates have become so used to sugary, over-processed foods that we crave them over those that heal us. Also, the marketing of over-processed foods – presented to us as treats and rewards – makes them more appealing, particularly if children are involved and the money available for food is limited. And, as we'll discuss in the next chapter, these foods are priced accordingly for over-consumption. The profit is based upon the fact that their lack of nutrition and negative impact on insulin levels (see next chapter) actually drives us back for more.

Foods high in fibre have the opposite effect: filling us up and keeping us satisfied until our body actually requires more food, not when manufacturers want us to have some.

PREVENT AND PROTECT

A final point. Fibre is not a cure, rather a vaccination. That is to say, a cure is treatment for when a condition becomes chronic, while a vaccination is a preventative measure that ensures you never get the condition in the first place.

In many ways, vaccinations are less celebrated than cures (COVID-19 notwithstanding); no one runs around shouting about how they never get the flu – but they would eulogise about a drug that stopped the symptoms once they'd caught it.

This may be another answer to the question: why has fibre fallen out of favour? Fibre has been going quietly about its business, protecting us from a range of potentially lethal conditions, ensuring we maintain a healthy weight and improving our well-being. But the lack of fanfare has meant it has slipped from our consciousness and our menus.

Fibre must take its rightful position as one of the most important substances we can use to support our health and longevity. Shout it from the rooftops: fibre is nature's vaccination.

Can you afford not to have it?

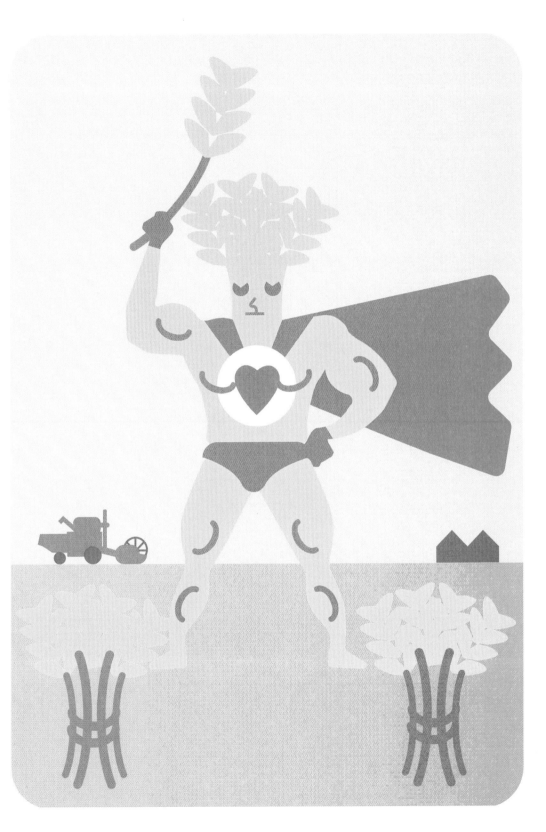

2. THE FIBRE CONS-PIRACY

'DAMNING SUGAR WILL NOT SOLVE OUR OBESITY PROBLEM – BUT CELEBRATING FIBRE WILL.'

efore we look at why fibre has been relegated to the lower nutrition leagues for the past couple of decades, let's get one thing out of the way: fibre has an image problem.

You know what I'm talking about; for most people when you mention fibre the first thing that springs to mind is a closed lavatory door and the hours spent sitting behind it. In the seventies and eighties fibre was synonymous with 'roughage'. Even today Germans refer to it as *Ballaststoffe* – weight matter – showing this bias. Despite the indisputable success of Audrey Eyton's *The F-Plan Diet* (Penguin) in the eighties, it left fibre with a reputation for being worthy, boring and, yes, lavatorial. The received wisdom about fibre is it fills you up, is a bit chewy and assists with regularity; the sort of thing that helps the infirm, not youthful people like us.

Thankfully, things have moved on and cutting-edge science on fibre is so exciting we really should be talking about it in terms of a health revolution, not as fusty old bran that you spoon on to your cereal in the mornings. The data on the benefits of increasing your fibre intake is quite overwhelming.

In truth, there are very few actual drugs for which we have a similar amount of data as we do for fibre, particularly as the science of the gut has evolved so much in the past decade. We now know so much more about our digestive system and the effect that it can have on our health and well-being. More importantly, its benefits put most medicines and health claims to shame.

The health industry obviously didn't get the memo as for years it has focused on fat, sugar and protein, and how much – or how little – we should be eating to maintain weight and general health. Because of this, fibre hasn't really been on the radar – or had a starring role in our menus – over the last forty years or so. Fad diets have come and gone at an alarming rate. Many – from the grapefruit diet or cabbage soup diet to low-carb, high-protein plans – are repackaged and relaunched every decade. There is nothing new about paleo or keto or the before-and-after pictures we are flooded with. People, however, seem to be waking up to the fact that they're ineffective and a waste of time. But what are the real solutions that actually work? Now is the right time for fibre to rejoin the discussion.

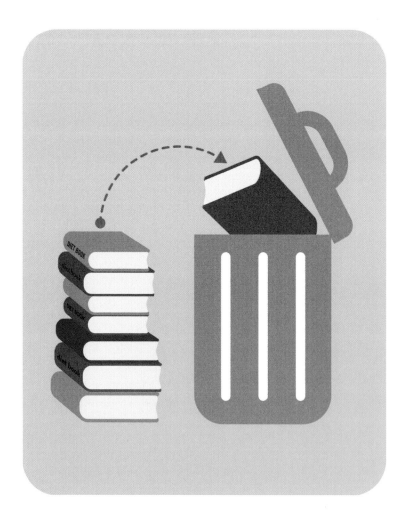

SPEED OF SUCCESS

If you look at the diet industry as a whole it has not succeeded; in fact, I think we can safely say that it has failed, miserably so. For the past thirty years, people have paid it vast amounts of money – to the tune of $450 billion per year – yet on a societal level we're more obese, overweight and unfit than we've ever been. Although the diet industry would say that this isn't their fault, if you look at meta-analyses the longer-term impact from diets is a meagre 3% weight reduction.[20] And this is for diets that are part of a structured programme with scientists following up, as opposed to the typical self-administered diet or diet plan.

Despite this obvious vigilance by the designers of the various studies, the drop-out rate is very high (about 25% per year). As a result, there are few reliable long-term studies of weight loss. To add insult to injury, about a third of people who diet regain more weight than they initially lose.[21] You can put anyone on a low-calorie diet and, if they stick to it, they'll lose weight. The problem is a diet needs to be sustainable over the long-term and the majority are the exact opposite.

The reason for this is simple: most diets require a lifestyle change that we are unwilling to commit to long term. We may think we are, but the data suggests otherwise. Under normal conditions, people on the whole do not change their lifestyle and that means that, even if we stop doing whatever it is that is making us obese for a short time, we will be pulled back into it. Not only that, but studies of the long-term outcomes of dieting show that most dieters will regain much of the weight they lost within twelve months and all of it within five years. It's very hard to escape both your own habits plus those imposed on you by your environment.[22] This, in my opinion, is the main reason diets don't work.[23]

The second reason is that people want a quick fix but this, too, is ultimately unsustainable. If you reduce your calories below a certain level, your metabolism adjusts to this new reality. This means that if you go back to the type of foods you ate before your diet intervention, your adjusted metabolism will cause the weight to pile back on. It is, therefore, not surprising that at least one third of people regain more weight than they lost. This has been observed in the majority of studies, but the root cause is not yet fully understood.[24]

There is almost an arms race for which diet can help you lose weight the fastest, but remember: the diet that takes away the weight quickest is the one that allows you to put it back on the quickest too.[25]

I've called this chapter 'The Fibre Conspiracy' because the data for fibre and against diets is so convincing one may, if so inclined, suspect foul play. Perhaps there's no evil intention from the diet industry. Maybe it's just the combination of an ever-evolving marketplace and the quick-fix demands of consumers that has led to an approach that favours restriction and the taking away of foods/ calories over a short period, rather than adding in the right nutrition over a longer period.

It'll be no surprise to you that my approach favours the latter. Fibre is not a quick-fix thing; it's for the long term. Critically, it does not require a lifestyle or significant menu change to achieve impressive results. And, far more important than obesity, it's actually fundamentally healthy in terms of the ability to prolong your life. Unfortunately for those chasing speedy results, you only notice your life getting longer over a lifetime, not over a matter of weeks.

MORE IS LESS

Another downside of the diet industry's demonising of certain food groups is the misinformation which now circulates about them. There are many diets that tell you to avoid carbohydrates, for example, but they don't specify which you should stay away from and which you should seek out.

Sugar and brown rice are both carbs, but they behave completely differently in the body. Sugar is classed as a simple carbohydrate and brown rice as a complex carbohydrate. Eat the same number of calories from each food and fundamentally different things happen in the body:

_____

+ Sugar gets absorbed immediately into the bloodstream, which is a sign for the pancreas to release insulin. This helps the blood sugar enter the body's liver, fat and muscle cells so it can be easily available as a source of energy or converted into fat. In the right amounts, sugar drives our metabolism and provides the short-term energy we need, but too much sugar, too often, can result in insulin resistance, which can lead to type 2 diabetes.

+ At a slightly simplified level, as our cells absorb the sugar and levels in our bloodstream begin to fall (and with it the insulin levels), the pancreas starts producing glucagon, a hormone that signals the liver to start releasing stored sugar, by promoting the breakdown of glycogen (stored sugar) to glucose in the liver, which then becomes available for the body to use. These two hormones play in tandem to ensure a steady supply of sugar for the organs to use.

+ The brain uses about 20–23% of the body's energy intake but, unlike other organs, it does not store much glycogen and pretty much only uses the glucose available in the blood. Any fall below a certain threshold will cause the brain to assume it is in starvation mode. The result is that you feel hungry (and hangry = hungry + angry), and a range of other symptoms such as dizziness, headaches, etc. – your brain is telling you to urgently get the next sugar hit.[26]

+ If we rely on sugary food to get us through the day – sugar-coated breakfast cereal, sweets and snacks, fizzy drinks – we end up see-sawing our way from one sugar rush to the next. The starvation mode is a powerful driver of our behaviour, which most of us know when we get irritable (or hangry) due to not having had food for a while. Our body is telling us to immediately forage or kill something to eat. Those of us who experience this state know that it is very difficult to resist eating that cookie sitting in front of us in the meeting room.

+ Alternatively, the very same amount of calories consumed in the form of complex carbohydrates, such as fibre-rich brown rice, will have a much smoother effect on your insulin response. Complex carbs release their sugars gradually, so you never really get to the insulin peak and trough and therefore your body doesn't crash and demand the next sugar hit. This modulation of the release of sugars has a huge effect on the way our overall consumption of calories happens. Fibre has a further impact by stretching out the happy phase of sufficient sugar availability.[27]

+ The well-known formula – calories in minus calories out equals weight gain or loss – is patently wrong because it ignores the impact of the nutrient, such as sugar, on our metabolism and the hormones involved. The same calories from sugar, fat, protein, complex carbs and fibre have fundamentally different effects on our metabolism and therefore on weight gain.

Eating sugary snacks throughout the day to satisfy dips in blood sugar will have a negative effect on weight management – but increase your fibre intake and you won't suffer those dips.

This is because fibre-rich foods also score highly on the satiety index: a scale developed to measure how satisfying foods are with regards to loss of appetite after eating. The index clearly shows the simpler the starches and sugars present in foods, the less satiating they are. The more fibre in the food – you guessed it – the longer it takes for you to feel hungry. [28]

Yes, protein also ranks high on the satiety index, but we're already eating too much: most adults need around 0.75g of protein per kg of body weight per day and in the UK (or the USA) we're eating double that. We really don't need any more. What we *do* need more of is fibre. And once you increase that in your diet, everything else falls into place.

You won't have to make any lifestyle changes or even consciously cut down on unhealthy foods. Simply choosing fibre-rich foods will reduce your cravings by modulating your blood sugar and making you feel fuller for longer. Eat more fibre and you'll automatically eat less, no diet required. Could this be why fibre has been kept off the table for so long? Maybe there is a conspiracy, after all…

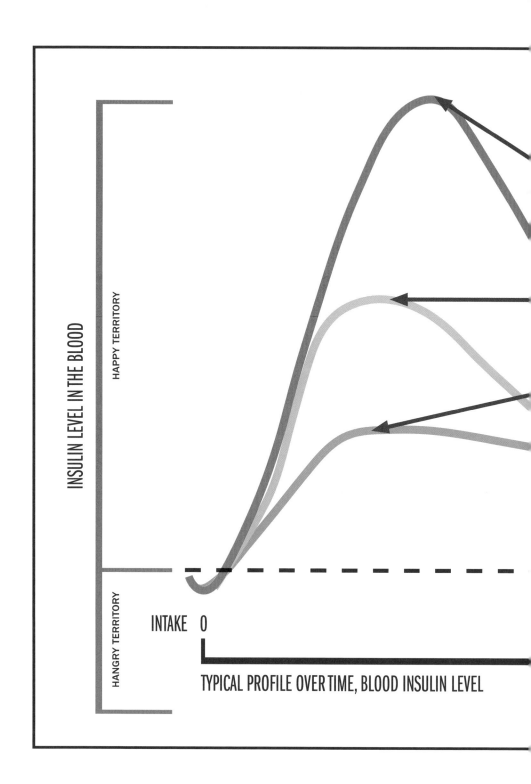

INSULIN LEVEL IN THE BLOOD

HAPPY TERRITORY

HANGRY TERRITORY

INTAKE 0

TYPICAL PROFILE OVER TIME, BLOOD INSULIN LEVEL

THE TYPE OF CALORIE YOU CONSUME MAKES A BIG DIFFERENCE ON YOUR METABOLISM

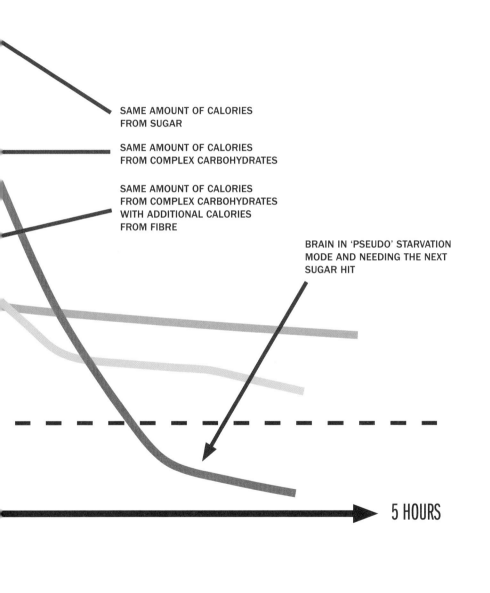

SAME AMOUNT OF CALORIES FROM SUGAR

SAME AMOUNT OF CALORIES FROM COMPLEX CARBOHYDRATES

SAME AMOUNT OF CALORIES FROM COMPLEX CARBOHYDRATES WITH ADDITIONAL CALORIES FROM FIBRE

BRAIN IN 'PSEUDO' STARVATION MODE AND NEEDING THE NEXT SUGAR HIT

5 HOURS

WHAT ABOUT GOVERNMENTS?

Let me pick an example of the utter failure to reduce sugar: Public Health England has overseen the government's strategy in reducing sugar and has published a report that shows, for example, that the introduction of a tax in 2017 on sugary drinks has led to a 28.8% fall in their sugar content (presumably replaced with sweeteners).[29] It also shows that for a basket of goods the sugar content has been reduced by 2.9% for in-home and 4.9% for out-of-home products (this is roughly the halfway point to a 2020 target of 20% reduction – in other words still a long way to go). The report celebrates the various achievements in reducing sugar in specific categories, but utterly fails to understand the gorilla in the room: the total sugar consumed went up by 2.6% from 2015–2019 according to the same report. In other words, we have rearranged the deck chairs on the obesity titanic. While I laud the fundamental intention to reduce obesity, especially in children, governments must wake up to the fact that their strategies are toothless at best and a waste of resources at worst.[30] The questions that must be answered are, why is the overall consumption of sugar going up despite the reduction in sugar in certain items? Is it because people simply consume more, or compensate for the lower amounts, say in reducing their soft drink consumption, by eating other sugary or energy-dense products such as cookies? Is it that replacing sugar with sweetener exacerbates the problem? Or is it that we continue to eat less and less fibre? I hope that I am proven wrong, but I will not hold my breath – especially since I believe there is a better, cheaper and more manageable solution.

SUBSTITUTING SUGAR WITH SWEETENERS DOES NOT SEEM TO BE A SOLUTION TO OUR OBESITY PROBLEM.

Recent studies (note, we do not yet have multiple meta-analyses to give us a high level of confidence) suggest that there may be one positive and two negative effects of sweeteners.

The positive effect is that non-caloric sweeteners do not cause an insulin response. This is, of course, significant as it cuts out an important mechanism for over-consumption.[31]

One negative effect seems to be that our brain (or gut-brain system) does not get fooled by sweetness that does not deliver calories, or potentially dissociates sweetness with the presence of calories. A result could be that we will over-consume other high-calorie products or compensate by eating other sugary products.[32]

Another negative effect seems to be the impact on our gut flora. Humans and mice fed on sweeteners seem to change their gut flora, and their ability to absorb sugar appears to increase significantly. In other words, our system simply adjusts by extracting sugar more efficiently, when we encounter it.[33]

This may be the explanation behind a number of studies that show that people on diet drinks or sweeteners not only do not lose weight, but are more obese than those who aren't exposed to sweeteners.

It is not clear at this point if there are differences between sweeteners[34] (all are used in minuscule amounts, except for sugar alcohols) and if the negative impact could be reversed, if sweeteners are consumed with some sugar and potentially also fibre.

More and more studies show that using sweeteners does not help reduce weight. They may even increase weight gain.[35]

FIBRE VERSUS PHARMA

In the previous chapter, I referred to fibre as a 'miracle drug'. I said that, in the future, we may look back over the past thirty years and wonder how we failed to notice its incredible health properties.

As we'll see in Chapter 6, it's easy to add fibre to popular dishes without changing flavour, texture or even cooking time. When I look at the data and how food is marketed, I can only surmise that people aren't doing this already and eating fibre-rich foods because a) they aren't aware of how powerful fibre is and b) it's been difficult to patent fibre and therefore harder to exploit on an exclusive commercial level.

A new drug enjoys patent protection and many years of high profits for its creators, but you couldn't treat, say, a raspberry in the same way. Raspberries are extremely high in fibre – one of the highest fruits – but how can you patent a berry?

There's also the fact that consuming different varieties of fibre sources together is healthier than any one specific type. They work in synergy. This makes it even more difficult for pharmaceutical companies to come up with a fibre product in their laboratories that they can patent for commercial purposes. They would need to show that their fibre product is better than naturally occurring fibre, which would be a time-consuming and costly process.[36] It's easier to sideline fibre and get on with promoting the commercial drugs.

And that is why we need to stand up for fibre and promote its health-giving properties in the same way a big pharmaceutical company would promote a new product. The effects really are that profound.

It's such an easy win: you don't have to change your lifestyle or stick to a diet, you just add more fibre – by stealth if need be – to what you and your family eat.

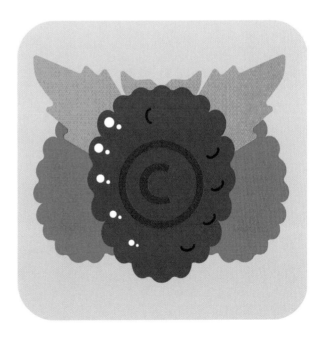

3. WHY FIBRE IS SO AMAZING

'THE MIRACLE THAT PUTS MOST MEDICINES AND HEALTH CLAIMS TO SHAME.'

S o what is fibre? In short, fibre is one of a group of macronutrients that we need to sustain life and maintain health. It's a carbohydrate – specifically a complex carbohydrate – that consists of long chains of sugar molecules. There are two types of chain linkages between the sugar molecules: those that our bodies can break down and those our bodies cannot. Complex carbohydrates, such as starches, take longer to be broken down, simply because they consist of very long and often branching chains. Simple carbohydrates are more easily broken down by our bodies as the chains are shorter. For example, granulated sugar is two molecules attached to each other: one glucose molecule and one fructose molecule. Our body can easily break those molecules apart and use them in its metabolism, but as more sugars are added the longer the chain becomes and the more difficult it is to break down.

Fibre, on the other hand, has links that cannot be broken down by us. There are two types of fibre: insoluble fibre and soluble fibre. Both pass through our upper intestinal tract (UIT) rather than being broken down (as simple carbs are), which means the sugar they contain does not get into our bloodstream.

Insoluble fibre passes through the human body without being broken down (some animals such as cows and other ruminants have very special digestive systems that are able to break it down). Its main function is to keep us full and bulk up stools, but it also appears to absorb some of the sugar we eat, preventing it from getting into our bloodstream in the UIT. This is roughly speaking the 'roughage' that was such a preoccupation of the high-fibre diets of the seventies and eighties.

Soluble fibre, on the other hand, does get broken down in our lower intestinal tract (LIT) by the microorganisms that live there. But rather than being absorbed into our bloodstream, the sugars released are quickly munched up by gut microbes – our 'friendly bacteria' that thrive on them. Without this soluble fibre, our friendly bacteria wither and our many body systems are negatively affected, ultimately shortening our lives.

A lot of the latest science focuses on the benefits of soluble fibre and, as this chapter is looking at nutrition and the gut, so will we, but that's not to sell insoluble fibre short.

It's also worth noting that different sources of fibre are preferred by different bacteria, so the wider range of fibre you eat, the better biodiversity you'll have in your intestine. As we'll see in Chapter 4, this is definitely a good thing.

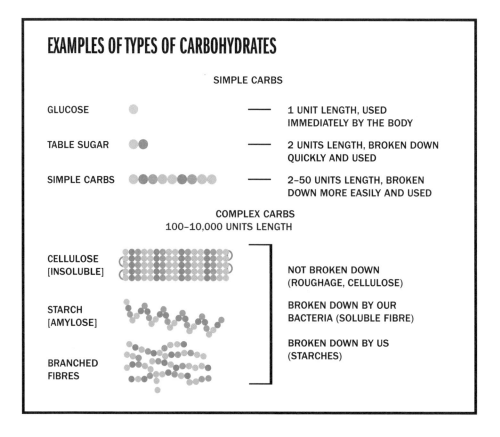

EXAMPLES OF TYPES OF CARBOHYDRATES

SIMPLE CARBS

GLUCOSE — 1 UNIT LENGTH, USED IMMEDIATELY BY THE BODY

TABLE SUGAR — 2 UNITS LENGTH, BROKEN DOWN QUICKLY AND USED

SIMPLE CARBS — 2-50 UNITS LENGTH, BROKEN DOWN MORE EASILY AND USED

COMPLEX CARBS
100–10,000 UNITS LENGTH

CELLULOSE [INSOLUBLE]

STARCH [AMYLOSE]

BRANCHED FIBRES

NOT BROKEN DOWN (ROUGHAGE, CELLULOSE)

BROKEN DOWN BY OUR BACTERIA (SOLUBLE FIBRE)

BROKEN DOWN BY US (STARCHES)

INSOLUBLE FIBRE

Unlike the soluble variety, insoluble fibre doesn't dissolve in water or gastrointestinal fluids when it enters our stomach and intestines. Rather it remains more or less unchanged as it moves through our digestive system.

Because it's not digested, insoluble fibre passes through our digestive system, absorbing fluid and adhering to other digestive by-products to form stools. In doing this, insoluble fibre speeds up the processing of waste and helps prevent constipation or any more serious gastrointestinal blockages, while ensuring we have healthy – and speedy – trips to the lavatory. This can also have a preventative effect on developing diverticular disease and even colorectal cancer.

Also, as insoluble fibre actually takes up physical space in the gut, it furthers the sensation of being full: a great ally with weight management.

NOT ALL CARBS ARE CREATED EQUAL

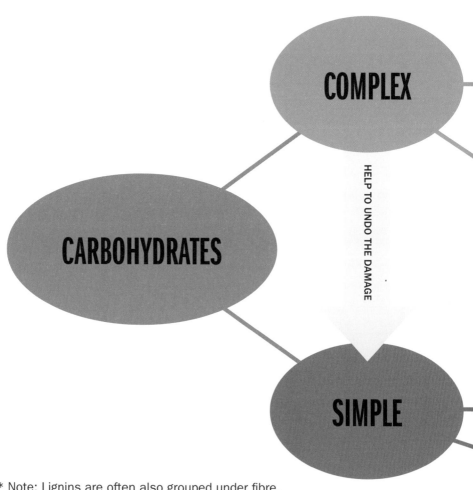

* Note: Lignins are often also grouped under fibre, but they are structurally different, and not fermented by our gut bacteria. They do have a minor benefit on how fermentable fibre is metabolised, but it is ignored in this context.

INSOLUBLE FIBRE
- Does not dissolve (roughage)
- Most cannot be fermented by our gut bacteria
- Can stimulate mucus formation in the intestines, thus creating bulking effect promoting regularity (e.g., psyllium)

FIBRE* — **SOLUBLE FIBRE**
- Ferments in the colon, food for our gut bacteria
- Some are viscous, creating feeling of fullness
- Binds bile acids and reduce cholesterol
- Some are non-viscous (dextrin, resistant starches, inulin)

COMPLEX CARBOHYDRATES
- Do not dissolve (roughage)
- Most cannot be fermented by our gut bacteria
- Can stimulate mucus formation in the intestines, thus creating bulking effect promoting regularity (e.g., psyllium)

SIMPLE STARCHES
- In a lot of processed foods
- Break down quickly into sugars
- Increase blood insulin levels

SUGARS
- Sweet taste
- Mostly glucose, fructose, lactose
- Increase blood insulin levels
- Increase cholesterol
- Increase obesity

There are a few sugar alcohols, notably Xylitol, that are metabolised by our gut bacteria and are prebiotic.

WHERE TO FIND FIBRE

Gone are the days of spooning bran on to your cereal to get your fibre fill – there are much tastier ways to enjoy the benefits.

As a rule, fibre is available in plant material, so anything that grows out of the ground will generally have some fibre in it (even mushrooms). However, not all plants are created equal and some plant material will have more fibre than others. This is often related to how much water it contains; for example, a large slice of watermelon is mostly water and very little fibre (0.4g fibre per 100g), whereas a handful of chia seeds has a lot of fibre (34g fibre per 100g). Generally, seeds and grains have 10–15% fibre per 100g and cooked lentils and pulses around 10%.

Then you have cooked nuts, which have the benefit of being 9–10% fibre as well as delivering some often very beneficial fats. Vegetables and fruit tend to be in the 4–5% range, with some, such as passion fruit, berries and avocado, almost twice that.

Interestingly, herbs such as mint, basil, coriander and rosemary are also quite high – around the 10% mark – but unfortunately in the Western diet we only tend to use them in small quantities to add flavour. In some cultures, such as my own Iranian culture, they are used more copiously, for example as a salad, maximising the fibre intake as well as other health benefits.

WHY SHOULD WE BE EATING FIBRE?

Fibre plays several roles when it comes to digestion. For a start, it bulks up our food and, as it passes through our digestive system, it binds a lot of water, increasing faecal weight and improving our regularity. While using the lavatory may not be something we want to dwell upon, regular and healthy trips to the loo are a very important part of weight management and general well-being.

The viscosity of some soluble fibres is also useful. Known as viscous fibres, they form a thick gel when they bind with water and then sit in the gut and slow down digestion and the absorption of nutrients, such as sugar and fat. They can bind to bile acids which can prevent a whole range of conditions. This viscosity assists with feelings of fullness and satiety, which in turn helps with weight management.

Then there are fermentable fibres which, unsurprisingly, are fermented by gut bacteria and increase bacterial mass and activity.

This fermentation is key to the production of short-chain fatty acids (SCFAs) which have various roles in the body, particularly in supporting our immunity by stimulating the production of immune system components, such as cytokines, leukocytes and helper T cells, and anti-inflammatory effects. There are a range of powerful effects that have been illuminated by science over the past decades that show the central role of these SCFAs. For example,

THE ROLES OF FIBRE

BULKING

+ Improves regularity by increasing faecal weight (because fibre binds a lot of water, e.g., coarse wheat bran), shortening transit time, and due to increase in bacterial mass (see fermentation)

VISCOSITY

+ Modulates sugar absorption
+ Modulates fat absorption
+ Impacts on bile acid absorption
+ Extends transit time in the gastrointestinal tract
+ Increases satiation (no longer having the desire to eat) and satiety (the feeling of fullness)

FERMENTATION

+ Feeds gut bacteria, increases bacterial mass and increases bacterial activity
+ Produces short-chain fatty acids which:
    + Have various effects on the body, particularly immunomodulation (e.g. stimulation of the production of immune system components, such as cytokines, leukocytes, helper T cells) and anti-inflammatory effects
    + Are an energy source for colonic cells/mucosa (butyric acid). Improve barrier properties of colonic mucosal layer and improve glucose absorption
    + Impact on bile acid metabolism and as a result on cholesterol metabolism (propionic acid)
    + Impact on pancreatic insulin and glycogen breakdown in the liver, thus stabilising glucose levels
    + Suppress cholesterol synthesis and reduce LDL (potentially also due to reduction of fructose load)
    + Increase acidity in the colon, thus protecting the lining and increasing the ability to absorb minerals and reduce formation of polyps
+ Traps bile acids
+ Increases intake of biologically active compounds (e.g., vitamins, minerals and phytochemicals)
+ Removes toxins
+ Synthesises vitamins (e.g., B, K)

SCFAs are an important energy source for colonic cells/mucosa (butyric acid). They improve barrier properties of the colonic mucosal layer and improve glucose absorption. They impact bile acid metabolism and, as a result, positively influence cholesterol metabolism (propionic acid). They have a direct impact on pancreatic insulin and glycogen breakdown in the liver, thus stabilising glucose levels. They also suppress cholesterol synthesis and reduce LDL (low-density lipoprotein) aka bad cholesterol levels.

Finally, being acidic, SCFAs increase acidity in the colon, thus protecting the lining and increasing the ability of the body to absorb minerals and reduce the formation of polyps. They also improve the lining of the gut and increase its ability to absorb minerals, metabolise bile acids and cholesterol, help break down glycogen and stabilise glucose levels and reduce LDL cholesterol.

VITAMINS AND DETOXING

Beyond the SCFAs, the soluble fibres and the bacteria that they feed help increase the intake of biologically active compounds (e.g., vitamins, minerals and phytochemicals), synthesise vitamins such as vitamin K and B vitamins, and help remove toxins through direct absorption by the fibre and the bacteria chewing on toxins and thus removing them before they reach our bloodstream. There are two detox systems in your body – your gut and your liver – so the next time you see an advert for a detox cure, just remember you have your gut already doing it for free.

And the benefits of bulking, viscosity and fermentation reach far beyond the gut.

The impact on metabolism can reduce the likelihood of pancreatic cancer, while improvements to the digestive system can reduce the incidence of inflammatory bowel diseases (IBD) and cancer of the bowel and oesophagus. By supporting the immune system and reducing inflammation (via SCFAs), fibre can support the respiratory system, reducing the severity of viral infections. It protects the cardiovascular system against coronary events, reducing stroke incidence, blood pressure and LDL cholesterol. There is strong evidence that increased fibre intake can reduce the risk of type 2 diabetes and there is emerging evidence for the reduced risk of a variety of cancers, including breast, uterus and kidney.[37]

On a lighter note, and as of yet not proven, the fact fibre improves mineral absorption means you might expect an improvement in the condition of your skin, hair and nails. Recent research demonstrates that higher fibre consumption is directly linked to the reduced rates of ageing at the chromosomal level due to inflammation and oxidative stress.[38] The benefits can be seen both inside and out.

HOW MUCH SHOULD WE BE EATING?

That we're not eating enough fibre is a given. The recommended average intake for an adult is 30g per day and many of us are barely getting half of that (about 18g per day). We'll talk more about what you can do in the kitchen to up your intake in the next chapter, but, as a guide, 15 additional grams roughly looks like any one of the treats below:

+ 300g fruit or vegetable (4 tomatoes, carrots or courgettes)
+ 50–100g seeds (handful of chia seeds)
+ 150g nuts (about 2 handfuls)
+ about 3 portions of porridge (120g)
+ a huge bowl of popcorn (about 100g) – my all-time favourite!

Or you can combine bits of each of the above to add to your daily meals: for breakfast some porridge with chia seeds and chunks of orange or apple; for lunch a big salad with steamed vegetables and roasted nut and seed crumble on top; and for dinner some quinoa and steamed vegetables next to other delicacies that you enjoy.

Now that may sound like a lot, particularly if your current intake is on the low end of the scale, but as we'll see you can easily boost your and your family's fibre intake by stealthily adding choice ingredients to established favourites.

If you don't want to trick your family (or yourself) into eating more fibre, you can simply look at the stark reality of the health benefits. There are probably more scientific studies and meta-analyses conducted on dietary fibre than any other natural compound. They all demonstrate the impressive benefits. For example, a recent meta-analysis commissioned by the WHO and published in scientific journal *The Lancet*, shows that for every additional 8g of fibre a day, risk of heart disease is reduced by 19%, risk of type 2 diabetes by 15%, risk of colon cancer by 8% and risk of all-cause mortality by 7%.[39] That should be enough to develop a taste for lentils.

You don't have to stop at 30g though: research suggests going beyond that amount further lowers your risk of all the chronic diseases we have talked about before, such as type 2 diabetes and heart disease.

As I mentioned in Chapter 1, this is the 'vaccination' side of fibre – the long game. In the short term, increasing your fibre intake will crowd out those bad nutrition choices that make weight management so difficult via greater satiety, reducing sugar and helping you ditch the junk food more easily. No diet required!

GAS PANIC!

Will I have to hide from the world every time I eat some fibre?

One hangover from fibre's seventies reputation is that too much can cause all sorts of digestive upsets including, most famously, uncomfortable bloating and wind. While I'm not going to say this isn't a possibility, particularly when starting out on a fibre-up journey, it's worth repeating that not all fibres are made the same, which, when coupled with our individual microbiomes, means that everyone's experience will be slightly different.

For example, my sister – and she won't thank me for telling you this! – can't eat chickpeas without suffering gas issues and yet I can eat them until the cows come home. Even though we have the same parents and grew up together, she has different bacteria to me and the way our microbiomes react to chickpeas is seemingly different.

Saying that, certain fibres, for example fructooligosaccharides such as inulin, are known to react with bacteria and create CO_2. They can be found in onions, garlic, Jerusalem artichokes, asparagus and leeks, and, while the resulting gas can be uncomfortable, it's not dangerous. However, people habituate, so even with those fibres that cause the most gas, over time (roughly a week) our microbiome will acclimatise to them. There may be a period of trial and error to see how you react to different foods, but again as individuals there's no set time limit. The fact of the matter is some foods, like beans, have a tendency to create gas, whereas others, like oats, don't. The best way to find out is to increase the diversity of what you eat and find out for yourself.

HYDRATION. IF FIBRE ABSORBS WATER, DO I HAVE TO DRINK MORE?

Another frequently asked question about upping fibre intake is whether it's wise to increase the amount of water you drink. Generally speaking, fibre in its natural form (fruit, vegetables and cooked grains or legumes) will already have a lot of water in it: we don't eat dry beans – we cook them in water first.[40] Fruit and vegetables are typically over 70% water; all the best sources of fibre come with water, so it's already hydrated so to speak.

If taking fibre supplements (see Chapter 5) – which I don't recommend as fibre is easily available from food – then it's important to ensure you drink enough water. Particularly with supplements where the fibre can gel, such as psyllium husk, because that can, in rare instances, cause issues such as clogging the oesophagus, which could be life-threatening.

PRE-EXISTING CONDITIONS. WHEN DO I HAVE TO WORRY ABOUT TAKING TOO MUCH FIBRE?

Even though fibre has a positive effect on the gut, for those who suffer from conditions such as irritable bowel syndrome (IBS), IBD, Crohn's and leaky gut it's best to be cautious. Often the root causes of such conditions are specific to an individual, but generally fibre should not hurt. However, there could be certain conditions where fibre would not be a good thing, particularly certain types of fibre, such as fructo-oligosaccharides that can promote gas. First talk to your doctor if you have any chronic problem, especially of the intestine, before significantly increasing your fibre intake.

4. UNDER-STANDING YOUR GUT

'FOR THE LOVE OF GUT, FEED THAT OCTOPUS.'

W e've talked a lot about how important fibre is for our gut. But why exactly, and what does it do when it gets there? Let's go right back to basics and take a quick and fascinating biology lesson.

US AND THEM

There are 100 trillion microorganisms, most of them bacteria, living in and on our bodies. That is about the number of stars in our galaxy or roughly one hundred times as many humans that have ever lived on Earth. Just think about that for a second: 100 *trillion*, all over your skin, in your mouth and, for the majority of them, in your gut; the large intestine to be precise. The bacteria (and a few other microorganisms) that reside in our gut collectively form our microbiome.

Now if you were brought up to fear bacteria and think of them as the root of all illness, then you might be feeling a bit concerned about there being 1–2kg of them living in the lower part of your gut. Particularly now, when antibacterial wipes and gels are part of our everyday life, shifting our mindset to think of bacteria as good for our health rather than bad is going to take some doing. But the fact remains, without bacteria we are nothing and we need to start thinking positively about them (at least most of them). You can almost think of our bodies as being inhabited by two beings: us and our healthy, friendly bacteria.[41]

DID YOU KNOW?

The surface area of the gut (32m^2) is the same as the surface of the roof of a bus – and about fifteen times greater than the entire surface of your skin.[42]

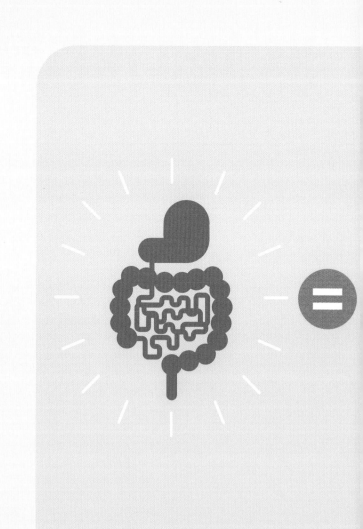

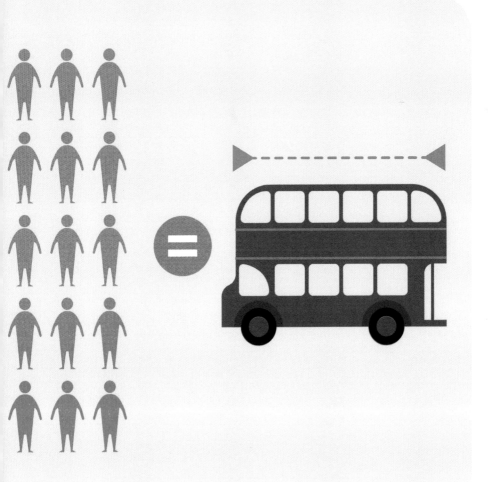

WHERE'S OUR MICROBIOME FROM?

When we're born we're basically sterile and without a microbiome. We get it from the very first bacteria we interact with: that of our mother. As a baby passes through the birth canal it's completely natural for it to come in contact with vaginal and faecal bacteria from its mother. It's these bacteria that are the building blocks of our microbiome.

The process is a little different for caesarean births as they obviously avoid the usual route, but a limited microbiome is still created from bacteria on the mother's skin and the hospital. Breastfeeding contributes further numbers to the burgeoning microbiome as the mother's milk acts as a powerful prebiotic to get the microbiome going.[43] Later on in life we have to shift to another prebiotic: fibre.

By the time we are two years old, our microbiome is classed as mature, although it's always shifting and changing as we're affected by a variety of external elements and microorganisms. These include our lifestyle, how much stress we're under or any medication we're taking. Even where we live can affect our microbiome; if you looked at the bacteria of someone who resides in a rural area and someone who lives in a city, they would be considerably different. But the biggest influence by far on our microbiome is how we feed it – and here's where fibre plays an essential role.

WHAT DOES OUR MICROBIOME DO?

That our microbiome is beneficial to our health and well-being is a given; it helps us in all sorts of ways – some we understand, some we don't yet. Nevertheless, it pays to start thinking of our gut bacteria as allies that need to be nurtured. If there's one thing us scientists are increasingly discovering, it's that if there's something wrong with the microbiome, then it will have a direct effect on a person's health. An imbalance in the gut bacteria can be the reason behind any number of ailments that affect our various body systems.

Everyone's microbiome may be unique, but the benefits of keeping it healthy are universal.

Let's start with what many people already know – better digestion, ensuring we get the most from the food that we eat and that what we don't require leaves our body as promptly as possible. From this comes more energy, better mood, healthier body systems, fewer illnesses and clearer thinking.

What is often not appreciated is that it's a self-perpetuating process: the better our digestion, the more diverse foods we can process; the greater the variety of nutrients we take on board, the greater the diversity of the bacteria that thrive in our gut; the more diverse our microbiome, the more efficient our digestion. And so on…

And it pays to keep our gut bacteria diverse. This is where our gut reveals its true health-giving power: it can protect us against pathogens; provide essential nutrients, enzymes and hormones; and train our immune system (the gut is the largest hormonal/endocrine organ in the body and makes up an important part of our overall immune system).[44]

Our gut bacteria help synthesise certain vitamins – notably vitamin K (good for bone health and wound healing) and a number of B-group vitamins (required for everything from energy to cell health to brain function) – and some amino acids (the building blocks of protein). Our gut bacteria also trap bile acids, increase the intake of vitamins, minerals and phytochemicals in our food, and help remove toxins. (If someone tries to sell you a detox snake oil, just tell them eating a carrot is more powerful and cheaper.)

They also produce important molecules that strengthen the lining of the gut, which stops bad bacteria getting through and causing problems with inflammation. One group of molecules called short-chain fatty acids (SCFAs), which we met in Chapter 3, act as powerful agents. They:

+ support our immune system
+ provide energy for colonic cells/mucosa
+ increase acidity in the colon, thus protecting the lining and increasing the ability to absorb minerals and reduce formation of polyps
+ metabolise bile acids and sterols, including cholesterol
+ help break down glycogen and stabilise glucose levels
+ reduce LDL (bad cholesterol)

HOW DOES A HEALTHY GUT PROLONG LIFE?

It's not just the health of our digestive system and the prevention of related diseases, such as IBS and IBD, that are linked to good gut health. Research has found links between a poor microbiome and a range of diseases. For some of these, the evidence is overwhelming and confirmed across many studies, while for others it is still tentative. In the strong evidence group you find some of the big killers:

+ cardiovascular diseases (coronary incidents, blood pressure, cholesterol, stroke)
+ colon cancer
+ pancreatic cancer
+ type 2 diabetes

THE CENTRAL ROLE OF FIBRE ON OUR BODY SYSTEMS

Strong evidence supported by meta-analyses, dose response

Good evidence supported by multiple studies, dose response relationship

Emerging evidence supported by multiple studies

Speculative based on a few studies but lacking convincing evidence

ENERGY/METABOLISM

- Reduce sugar absorption
- Reduced pancreatic cancer incidence
- Reduced inflammation

DIGESTIVE SYSTEM

- Reduced bowel cancer incidence
- Impact on inflammatory bowl diseases
- Reduced cancer of the oesophagus incidence
- Reduction of constipation

IMMUNE SYSTEM

- Immunomodulation and reduction of inflammation (including ageing)

RESPIRATORY SYSTEM

- Reduction of severity and time of lung viral infections (flu, COVID-19)
- Reduced COPD

BRAIN

- Reduced ADHD incidence (potentially indirectly due to lowering of fat and sugar)
- Reduction of depression and anxiety

BONES, SKIN, HAIR, NAILS

- Higher mineral absorption

CARDIOVASCULAR SYSTEM ENERGY/METABOLISM

- Reduced cardiovascular disease
- Reduced coronary events
- Reduced stroke incidence
- Reduction of LDL cholesterol
- Reduction of blood pressure

OTHER

- Reduces type 2 diabetes
- Reduced breast cancer incidence
- Reduced kidney/renal cancer incidence
- Reduced uterus/ovarian cancers incidence
- Reduced prostate cancer incidence

For the latest visit www.fiber4life.com

This is also the fundamental reason why fibre adds years to your life; it simply prevents these killers from getting to you.

In the more tentative group you find:

+ breast cancer
+ cancers of the kidneys, uterus, oesophagus
+ respiratory tract diseases (e.g. COPD)

And finally in the speculative group you find a wide range of claims, some of the more promising ones are:

+ depression
+ anxiety
+ ADHD
+ beauty and ageing

Let's be clear, it's not always a straightforward cause-and-effect situation, but rather because the gut is where a significant part of our immune system resides and where much of inflammation begins, any issues or imbalances there increase the likelihood of developing such conditions – preventing these conditions is preferable to trying to cure them.

There are links between gut health and weight management too. Our gut microbiome is involved in metabolism and can alter how we store fat, balance our blood sugar and respond to hormones indicating hunger and satiety. With the right mix, everything works as it should and we don't overeat or have problems with insulin; the wrong mix and we could be in the running for obesity and type 2 diabetes.

The good news is you can change your microbiome, and quickly too. And there are no prizes for guessing what's at the top of the list of foods you need to eat more of to do so.

OUR SECOND BRAIN: THE SMARTER YOU

We've all used phrases such as 'gut reaction', 'gut-wrenching' and 'feeling gutted', and for good reason, because there's a very real relationship between our gut and our emotions. Known as the brain–gut axis, it explains how our feelings can affect our digestion (and vice versa). It should come as no surprise that there are 500 million neurons surrounding the gut, the largest number outside of the brain and the spinal column. This group of cells are called the enteric nervous system and they link our central nervous, immune and digestive systems. The size of this second brain is the same as that of an octopus.

When the Sea Star Aquarium in Coburg, Germany, added Otto the octopus to its collection, little did they know that this smart creature would make some of them believe in ghosts. For a number of nights in a row the entire electrical system of the aquarium would short out. It took a few of the staff keeping a 24-hour vigil to discover that Otto was having fun climbing up from his enclosure and squirting water on to the spotlights overhead. Just for fun. Otto is not alone. Octopi have been observed sabotaging their tanks, escaping in ingenious ways, solving complex problems and forming bonds with people. Our gut brain may be in the same league as an octopus's brain and we better make friends with it or it can easily sabotage us.

Everything from butterflies in our stomachs when excited, to frantic toilet trips when nervous, shows that one of the avenues our brain utilises to express itself is the gut. But it's not a one-way street; research now points to the gut having a similar ability to affect our mental acuity, which is why our gut is sometimes referred to as our 'second brain'.

How this 'octopus' works is still a bit of a mystery even to us scientists, but we do know there's a lump of neurons sitting around our gut sending signals back and forth to our brain. What we also know is that, if we feed this 'octopus' correctly, then the positive outcomes in different body systems are profound.

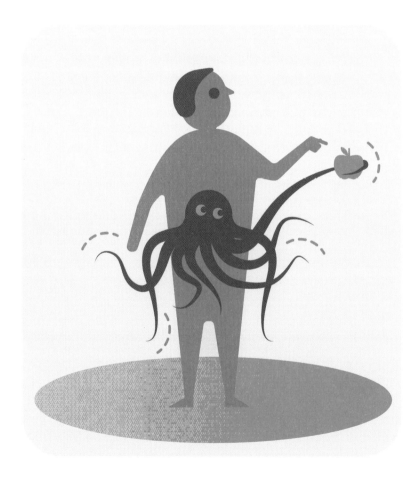

WE'RE IN CONTROL

The good news is that we can affect change in our microbiome in a relatively short space of time. Microbes renew every twenty minutes or so, which means that if we start giving our healthy gut bacteria what they need to do their job properly, they will adapt very quickly.

If our diets are deficient in fibre, it stands to reason that our microbiome will be deficient in the bacteria that fibre promotes. Luckily our microbes adapt to the food we give them. A 2017 study of the Hadza people of Tanzania found that those among them who lived as hunter-gatherers had a microbiome that reflected the seasonal nature of their diet.[45] At some points in the year, say when they were eating mainly meat, certain bacteria almost disappeared from their microbiome, only to reappear again when their diet seasonally shifted to a more plant-based phase.

A comparison was made with a more Westernised diet which also found certain bacteria lacking, but unlike the seasonal cycling of the Hadza people, the microbiome didn't change.

DIVERSITY, DIVERSITY, DIVERSITY

Any restrictive diet you go on will reduce the diversity of the food you eat and have a negative effect on your microbiome. A processed, limited diet, high in sugar, that suppresses beneficial bacteria and allows unhealthy strains to proliferate, is just as restrictive as the Paleo, low-carb or any other elimination diet you can think of. These diets don't just starve the body, they starve the gut too.

We are denying our microbiome the variety of nutrients it needs to flourish and, in doing so, we're denying ourselves far-reaching benefits for all aspects of our health – not just improved digestion but improvements to weight management, our immune system, cardiovascular system, and lowering risk of some cancers and potentially even depression.

Sure, we can survive on our current diet, but there's a big difference between surviving and *thriving*.

In short, your gut microbiome is key to your health. The greater the variety of food (read fibre) you eat, the greater the variety of bacteria you'll develop. Studies show an abundant and diverse microbiome is linked to greater health and well-being and reduced risk of everything I talked about above.

And the bacteria that make up your microbiome just love fibre, they munch it up. The more fibre you can give your 'octopus' the more abundant the microbiome will be. The more different types of fibre you can give it, the more diverse your microbiome will be.

OUR GUT DÆMON

I like to compare our gut to the dæmons in Philip Pullman's *His Dark Materials* trilogy: these dæmons are a manifestation of our true selves, a kind of spirit animal. In the fantasy world of Pullman the dæmons are beings that exist outside your body and follow you around. If separated from their dæmon, a person is blank and lifeless, with reduced creativity, intelligence and willpower. The same can be said of us if disconnected from our gut: it's our ally and keeps us healthy. If our gut was an external animal we'd want to look after it and feed it correctly, not give it food that would make it unwell and miserable. It's our responsibility to give our internal dæmon what it needs. And what it needs is fibre.

Just to rub it in: you would be shocked if you found out that your good friend, Jack, was starving his dog and feeding the poor thing nachos and lettuce because he keeps forgetting to buy dog food. You would get very angry, call the authorities or adopt the dog, if he would not change his ways. Jack is a pretty good characterisation of most of us and the next chapter will show easy ways to get Jack back on track.

5. THE FIBRE FIX: WHAT YOU NEED TO EAT

'THE DIET TO END ALL DIETS.'

By now you know what fibre is, what it can do for you and where you can get it from. But how does that translate into real life? It's all very well knowing that you should be getting at least 25–30g of fibre in your diet every day. But what does that look like when you're having a busy day at work or eating out in the evening?

This chapter will show you how to base your food choices on not just what's tasty for your palate but what's nutritious for your gut, too. Remember the dæmon or our friendly octopus from the previous chapter? Well, it still needs looking after, so let's find out how.

ISN'T HEALTHY FOOD EXPENSIVE?

Before we get to that though, let's just clear one thing up. There's a misconception that high-fibre foods – and healthy foods in general – are more expensive than more processed foods.[46] Sure, if you shop at some of the more top-end health food shops, expect to pay a premium. But for the most part, fibre-based alternatives to what are regarded as 'junk foods' are no more expensive, particularly when measured in terms of satiety as opposed to portion sizes. Who has ever binged on brown rice?

A quick comparison between 'junk foods' and their high-fibre counterparts (see pages 94–5) shows that our fibre friends are comparable in price, even a little cheaper. But if we switch that comparison to the cost per gram of fibre, we soon see that to get the health-giving benefits, you'll have to pay a whole lot more for your junk food than for your fibre-rich foods. So, despite some people's misconception, there's no evidence high-fibre grains or vegetables are expensive items.

FIBRE AND FIBRE-CONTAINING PRODUCTS ARE NOT MORE EXPENSIVE THAN JUNK FOOD

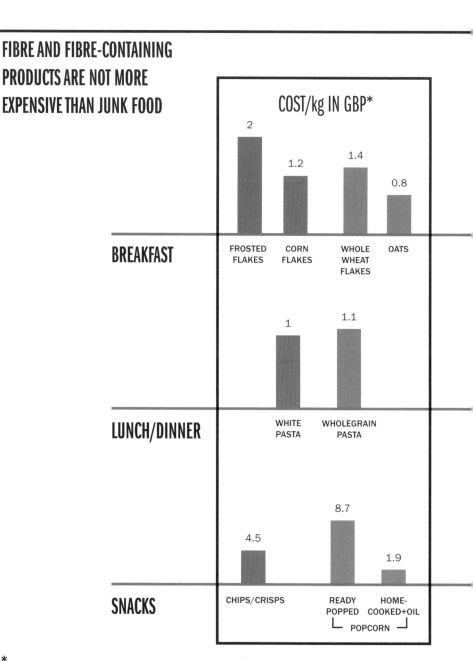

COST/kg IN GBP*

BREAKFAST

2 — FROSTED FLAKES
1.2 — CORN FLAKES
1.4 — WHOLE WHEAT FLAKES
0.8 — OATS

LUNCH/DINNER

1 — WHITE PASTA
1.1 — WHOLEGRAIN PASTA

SNACKS

4.5 — CHIPS/CRISPS
8.7 — READY POPPED POPCORN
1.9 — HOME-COOKED+OIL POPCORN

*Lowest prices available at UK's largest retailer (same day)
I tried to be fair here and not shop for the lowest price across many retailers or items on promotion. The above data comes closest to what a shopper experiences in a store or on line. For example, I could easily find wholegrain pasta at less than 0.8 GBP/kg instead of the 1.1 quoted here when shopping around.

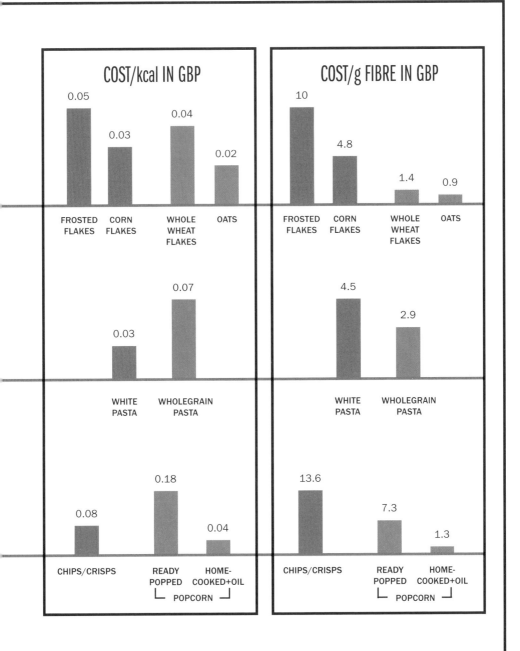

COST/kcal IN GBP

FROSTED FLAKES 0.05
CORN FLAKES 0.03
WHOLE WHEAT FLAKES 0.04
OATS 0.02

WHITE PASTA 0.03
WHOLEGRAIN PASTA 0.07

CHIPS/CRISPS 0.08
READY POPPED 0.18
HOME-COOKED+OIL 0.04
└ POPCORN ┘

COST/g FIBRE IN GBP

FROSTED FLAKES 10
CORN FLAKES 4.8
WHOLE WHEAT FLAKES 1.4
OATS 0.9

WHITE PASTA 4.5
WHOLEGRAIN PASTA 2.9

CHIPS/CRISPS 13.6
READY POPPED 7.3
HOME-COOKED+OIL 1.3
└ POPCORN ┘

SUGAR-TO-FIBRE RATIO: A REMINDER

As I talked about in Chapter 1, on a societal level, the sugar-to-fibre ratio is the best metric for improving a nation's health, without taxing its economy. The per capita spending on obesity, for example, directly reflects the sugar-to-fibre consumption of a country, meaning the more fibre a nation eats compared to the amount of sugar, the better its societal health and the healthy longevity of its citizens.

Some things, however, are easier said than done. We may now be aware that we need more fibre, but our palates have become so used to sugary, over-processed foods that we crave them over foods that actually do us good.

Luckily, there's an easy way to ensure you stay sugar-to-fibre aware, whether out and about or at home in your own kitchen. And that way is the 'Fibre Rule of Thumb'.

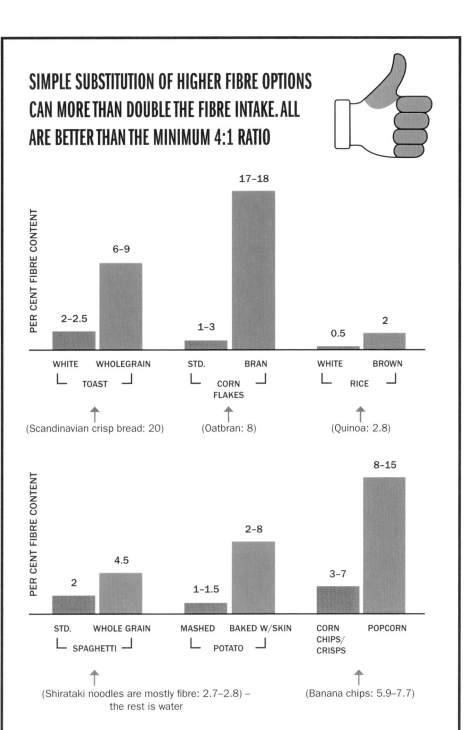

SIMPLE SUBSTITUTION OF HIGHER FIBRE OPTIONS CAN MORE THAN DOUBLE THE FIBRE INTAKE. ALL ARE BETTER THAN THE MINIMUM 4:1 RATIO

PER CENT FIBRE CONTENT

17–18

6–9

2–2.5

1–3

0.5

2

WHITE | WHOLEGRAIN
⌞ TOAST ⌟

STD. | BRAN
⌞ CORN ⌟
FLAKES

WHITE | BROWN
⌞ RICE ⌟

(Scandinavian crisp bread: 20)   (Oatbran: 8)   (Quinoa: 2.8)

PER CENT FIBRE CONTENT

8–15

4.5

2

1–1.5

2–8

3–7

STD. | WHOLE GRAIN
⌞ SPAGHETTI ⌟

MASHED | BAKED W/SKIN
⌞ POTATO ⌟

CORN | POPCORN
CHIPS/
CRISPS

(Shirataki noodles are mostly fibre: 2.7–2.8) –
the rest is water

(Banana chips: 5.9–7.7)

MY TOP TEN HIGH-FIBRE FOODS

1   **Seeds** (15%)

2   **Grains** (13%)

3   **Lentils, cooked** (10%)

4   **Herbs** (many have around 10%)

5   **Nuts** (9%)

6   **Legumes**, e.g. cooked beans, peas, legumes and raw peanuts (9%)

7   **Berries** (7%)

8   **Vegetables** (7%).

9   **Root vegetables** (5%)

10   **Fruit** (4%); avocados and passion fruit have around 9%

MY PERSONAL TOP TEN HIGH-FIBRE INGREDIENTS TO SNEAK INTO MY FOOD

1 **CHIA, SESAME AND FLAX/LINSEEDS (27%)**
I sprinkle them on everything. Chia seeds also make a great porridge.

2 **BARLEY (17%)**
Very versatile. Use in porridge, soup or as a side dish. I like that it is not so gooey.

3 **POPCORN (15%)**
Movie time. But I always pop it myself.

4 **ALL HERBS (7-40%)**
Parsley, sage, rosemary and thyme (and mint). I add them to everything.

5 **ALMONDS (12%)**
I munch them all the time, especially smoked.

6 **BUTTER BEANS (12%)**
More than twice the fibre of edamame beans, but prepared the same way.

7 **ARTICHOKES AND LEEKS (10%)**
Into the oven wrapped in foil – out comes heaven.

8 **AVOCADOS (9%)**
My go-to butter and I love guacamole.

9 **PASSION FRUIT (9%)**
Only sweet ones – when they are good they are magical.

10 **RASPBERRIES (8%)**
I can't get enough. They show up in my sauces, salads, cereal or just straight.

Whether out shopping or buying online, looking for a quick snack or planning a family meal, use the Fibre Rule of Thumb to ensure that what's in your shopping basket is giving you the optimum fibre bang for your sugar buck.

The minimum sugar-to-fibre ratio is 4:1; that's four parts of sugar to one part of fibre. Just use your hand to remind you: four fingers of sugar to one thumb of fibre. Any more fingers added is a bad trend. Of course there are going to be the occasional ingredients, condiments and treats that won't adhere to this rule – personally I can't live without my dark chocolate (six fingers to one thumb ratio), but as long as in the wider scheme of things these treats remain exactly that – treats for special occasions – then there's no harm done. Remember, this isn't a diet, just a way of maintaining vigilance and being aware of keeping your fibre intake at a better ratio than four sugars to one fibre.

SHOPPING LISTS

It's all well and good having me explain to you why you should be eating fibre, but how does it translate to the real world when supermarket shopping or ordering online? The answer is a good old-fashioned shopping list.

While I don't claim that they are complete, the lists on the following pages give you a good selection of readily available foods that are high in fibre and will go some way towards your 30g+ a day. Some items on the list may already be nestling away in your fridge, while others may be new to you. What they all offer are the benefits of a high-fibre diet along with an array of vitamins, minerals and phytonutrients.

STORE CUPBOARD

Seeds (15%) – mostly to sprinkle on foods or as part of
breakfast muesli or granola

+ sesame and nigella (give a savoury/moorish flavour)
+ pumpkin and sunflower (taste great when roasted)
+ flax and chia (not much taste, so can be easily
added to anything, even drinks)

Grains (13%)

+ whole oats (great for making porridge or muesli)
+ buckwheat (great for porridge or muesli, remember to
soak it first in water to get rid of an irritant, great for
people who don't want gluten)
+ wholewheat (perfect for breads, especially if you're
into sourdough)
+ wholegrain rye (tasty grain for baking)
+ spelt (an ancient grain dating back to the Bronze
Age, excellent for making bread)
+ amaranth (easy to cook with and behaves a bit like
semolina, can also be popped like popcorn)
+ quinoa (high protein – substitute for rice)
+ rice (ideally brown or black), wild rice (which is very
high in fibre, about 25%)
+ millet (has been around for the past 10,000 years
and packs lots of protein, fibre and calcium)
+ whole barley (works well in soups)
+ corn and popcorn

Nuts (9%)

+ almonds and almond butter
+ walnuts (if you let them sit in slightly salted water
overnight in the fridge, they will amaze you, crunchy
and a delight to put on salads or in sandwiches)

Legumes, e.g. cooked beans, peas, legumes and raw
  peanuts (9%)
+ baked beans
+ runner beans, broad beans, kidney beans, butter
  beans, haricots, cannellini beans, flageolet beans,
  pinto beans, borlotti beans (again dried or tinned)
Lentils and peas (cooked) (10%)
+ red, yellow, green, brown and Puy lentils
+ chickpeas, green peas, black-eyed peas
Dried fruit, especially prunes and dates (both are great
  for sweetening dishes)
Alliums
+ onions (I could not live without them)
+ garlic

FREEZER (often better than fresh as the product
is frozen at source and doesn't lose some of
its vitamins on the way to the shops – and is
more affordable!)

Fruit
+ avocados
+ berries (blueberries, raspberries)
+ mangos
Legumes
+ French beans, peas
Herbs
+ tarragon, mint, coriander, dill, basil
Vegetables (often you can buy mixes, great for stews
  and fried vegetable dishes)
+ spinach
+ carrots
+ broccoli and cauliflower

FRIDGE

Fruit (except for bananas, all others benefit from being in the fridge)
+ avocados (nature's butter and of course the main ingredient for guacamole – see recipe on page 129)
+ all citrus (my favourite are pomelos, the largest of all citrus fruits. Surprisingly the thick skin can be soaked for a few days to get rid of the bitter taste and then used as a vegetable or to make jams – very high in fibre.)
+ fresh almonds (with the outer skin intact and before the shell hardens. You can eat the whole thing – great as a snack, just sprinkle with a bit of salt not unlike edamame beans.)

Herbs (generally don't keep well and you could freeze any unused portion). They give excellent taste to any dish, but you can also make a salad from them, which will be the highest fibre salad you have ever had: basil (sweet, Thai), parsley, chives, mint, tarragon and coriander are my favourites

Vegetables
+ broccoli
+ butternut squash
+ celery
+ courgettes
+ peppers (red, yellow, green)
+ pumpkin
+ sprouted seeds

Roots (great for roasting)
+ carrots
+ celeriac
+ swede
+ yams and sweet potato

+ leeks
+ ginger and galangal (they just elevate any dish)
Pulses (eat raw or as part of a stew or steamed)
+ French beans
+ mangetout
+ peas

FRUIT BOWL

It is always great to have one to entice you to snack during the day. I have included those that tend to keep longer.

+ apples
+ bananas
+ kiwi fruit
+ oranges
+ lemons and limes (great for giving zing to dishes and salads)
+ passion fruit (very high in fibre)
+ papaya
+ peaches and nectarines
+ plums

SNACK SWAPS

Snacking is an opportunity for increasing fibre and helping you avoid making bad food choices when ravenous, so it's always a good idea to keep a high-fibre option in your glove compartment, drawer at work, handbag and so on. In my case, together with a piece of chocolate! If you have the satiating fibre-snack first, you won't need much of the chocolate, and it won't do any harm.

The obvious alternatives to nutritionally poor snacks are items such as fruit and nuts, both of which will go towards increasing your fibre intake. You could choose nuts, such as walnuts and almonds, which are great with high-fibre oatcakes, or sliced fruit or hummus with vegetable crudités or oatcakes. Shop-bought variants of the above are fine, but if you're feeling adventurous you could make your own, adding a handful of seeds to boost the fibre content further, plus you'll be cutting out any surreptitious sugar (believe me – it's in everything).

Even when looking at unhealthy products, such as ice cream, and then selecting those that claim to be better alternatives, you can see a huge difference between the options offered in the market. This just shows that with a little bit of scrutiny and searching, you can find commercial products with superior health value (and of course taste).

And for those with a penchant for crisps and savoury snacks, I can recommend popcorn as an alternative. A healthy wholegrain, its fibre content can be anything up to 15% and if you pop your own rather than buying ready-made, it can be a viable alternative to high-fat, low-fibre potato crisps.

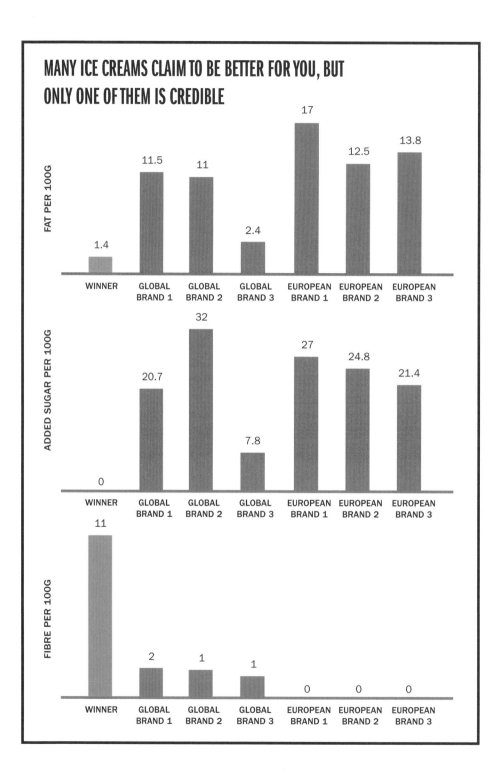

MANY ICE CREAMS CLAIM TO BE BETTER FOR YOU, BUT ONLY ONE OF THEM IS CREDIBLE

MY ANTI-DIET PLAN

Any diet that expects something from us is not going to work. There's only so much willpower to go around and for most people that's taken up by children, work and relationships. While there are incentives that can redirect our willpower at certain times – I used to exercise a lot more when I was dating – the moment the parameters change we tend to fall back into comfortable patterns. It's unfortunate, then, that most diets do expect something from us, and usually that involves cutting back on things we enjoy.

This is not a diet book, but I do have a plan you can follow. It doesn't require you to cut back on anything or stop doing something you enjoy. All it requires is that you pay a bit more attention to what you're eating when it comes to fibre content. Sounds simple? That's because it is! Before delving further into my ideas, let's first take a step back and see what problems we are trying to solve:

+ People have a hard time adjusting their lifestyle. Despite the well-known health issues with sugar, substitution with non-caloric sweetener and governments taxing it, sugar consumption and obesity continue to rise.
+ We chronically do not eat enough fibre.
+ We gain weight for three main reasons:

1. We overeat all macronutrients except for fibre. This means that our metabolism doesn't behave at its optimum level and we're more prone to hunger pangs, particularly when consuming simple sugars.

2. We eat everything on our plates because we don't notice when we are full (by the time our gut signals to the brain that it is full, we have long finished our plate – just remember the last meal where you slumped back in your chair, held your belly and exclaimed, 'Oh my god, did I overeat this time!').

3. We don't move enough and often don't get enough sleep.[47]

Any diet must address the points above or it will not work in the long run. My four-stage Anti-Diet Plan starts slowly and at each stage adds a subtle shift; even Stage 3 involves far less than most popular diets demand. It is designed in such a way that you can move from stage to stage (up or down the levels) always staying at where you are enjoying your life and do not feel that you are giving up pleasure. It combines the latest science on what keeps us healthy (remember healthy longevity is the goal) based on nutrition, physical activity and motivation (especially getting enough sleep) and uses psychological nudges to put you in the driver's seat. No need for a guru, gadgets or fairy tales to make you part with your hard-earned money. The before and after picture is simply you, giving yourself years of enjoyable life, and spending the money you save on diets on yourself and your loved ones.

My plan doesn't make any unrealistic promises; instead it aims to help you find out for yourself the benefits of increasing your fibre intake, while giving you a structure to take your fibre journey further if you so wish, by using the recipes in Chapter 6. Remember, this plan is not prescriptive. It's a guide to help ease you into thinking about fibre in relation to what you do already. There's no time limit for each level – this is an exercise in awareness not dogma. Remember my promise at the beginning of the book: this is about more fibre, not less enjoyment.

FIBRE-UP IN STAGES: MY ANTI-DIET PLAN

YOUR STATUS-QUO: HAPPY-GO-LUCKY

This stage focuses on your enjoyment and self-awareness.

+ Keep going as before. Who cares about dieting? Just enjoy your life and as long as you are happy with your health (not body shape), keep on rocking. All you want to do is to reflect on your current state:

  + What dishes do I particularly enjoy? Why?
  + What did I enjoy as a kid? Do I still enjoy it?
  + Which fruits and vegetables do I like? Why?
  + Is there any bird food that I like (e.g. nuts, seeds)?
  + What amount of food is sufficient to fill me up?

+ When you eat anything ask yourself if you are actually enjoying it or if there is a way to make that food more enjoyable:

  + better ingredients
  + less or more of something

+ We all love sweet things and our tongue is a powerful detector for sugar (most people can detect sugar at 0.05% levels; diabetics are less sensitive).[48]

+ Notice where you detect sugar when you eat a store-bought snack, drink or food or when you are eating a meal at a restaurant (just use your tongue as a detector).
+ Do you actually like the foods with a sweeter taste?

+ Think about what type of physical activity you enjoy or are good at. Why?

+ At night when you're about to fall asleep try this fun exercise: Ask yourself, which part of your body sends the strongest signal at that moment in time. It could be a sense of warmth, a little pain, an itch or simply where your thoughts end up. Stay in that focus and see if anything develops. If you can reach that spot, place your hand on it. This simple exercise tends to focus people inwards and into the body and reduce the cacophony of thoughts, which are essential during the day but can be an impediment at night.

STAGE 1: FIBRE IS FUN

This stage focuses on subtle nudges and increasing pleasurable experiences.

+ Have about 2.5g fibre 20–40 minutes before a meal (about a handful of sunflower seeds or almonds, a banana or an orange). This is to ensure that satiety signals get to your brain before you start your meal.

+ Eat to your heart's desire, and further develop awareness on the questions in Your Status Quo:

  + Now that you are eating less and spending less money, can you shift things to higher quality or higher pleasure dishes or ingredients?
  + What foods do you celebrate with (for me it is chocolate with hazelnuts)? Are there any that are better than others?

+ Set your phone to blue light filter or night mode to help with getting tired at night. Low amounts of sleep tend to reduce our ability to stick to our plans, and many compensate by eating energy-dense comfort foods.

STAGE 2: THE BALANCED LIFE

This stage brings together food, physical activity and sleep in a fun and easily implementable way.

+ Have 5g fibre 20–40 minutes before a meal (this is about 2 handfuls of sunflower seeds or walnuts, 2 bananas or 2 oranges). Eat your favourite foods, but substitute higher fibre versions (e.g. wholegrain, bran, whole fruit, etc.). See the suggestions in Chapter 6.[49]

+ Look at where you can increase your physical activity without much effort or going out of your way (e.g. walk up the stairs, walk to the shops, ride your bike, get the dog you always wanted). Think of it like brushing your teeth: it doesn't have to be something you pay much attention to, but you make sure it gets done, every single day! About 10 minutes of additional moderate activity a day is all that you need to do at this stage.[50]

+ When you decide to sleep, use the '7 x 7' technique to calm things down: breathe in slowly counting to seven (over seven seconds) and breathe out slowly counting to seven.[51] If this doesn't work for you, try the 'Rhythm and Blues' technique: lie in your bed and tap your body (thigh, arm, stomach, whatever feels comfortable) with your hand at a certain comfortable rhythm (typically one beat every second). After about a minute reduce the rhythm gradually.[52] Both of these techniques need a little practice – when you do the 7 x 7 you can find that you count too fast or get a little out of breath; for the Rhythm and Blues technique your hand might get tired. Don't worry, it's part and parcel of the method.

STAGE 3: FIBRE-UP

This stage is basically the same as Stage 2, with just a bit more effort.

+ Snack on fibre five times a day (2.5g each time). The only requirement is to keep snacks to a 4:1 ratio of sugar to fibre and drop this gradually to 1:1:

    + before breakfast (unless you are eating a fibre-full breakfast, such as muesli, granola, wholegrain bread, fresh fruit, etc.)
    + mid-morning
    + before lunch
    + mid-afternoon
    + before dinner

+ In addition to eating your fibre-up favourite foods, consider swapping out other fibre-containing ingredients (e.g. quinoa for brown rice, shirataki noodles for wholegrain noodles, more raw vegetables, sweeten dishes with whole fruit).

+ Normally, the high level of fibre will automatically reduce your portion sizes; however, you can try and use smaller plates (the size should be such that you feel full but not over-full) to further encourage yourself to eat until happy but not more.

+ Don't forget to reward yourself with something naughty but small at the end of a meal (we tend to remember the last thing we do more vividly).

+ Find ways of reducing added sugar in the smallest increments. It took me 2 years to go from 2 spoonfuls of sugar in my coffee to none. I went from 2 spoonfuls to actually using my finger to properly get a spoonful by removing the excess mountain, then by flicking a little away, then a spoon-and-a-half – you get the point.

+ Try to do some cardio exercise every day. Anything that gets your heart pumping: chasing your pet or your kids, simple push-ups, running upstairs, heavy gardening, doing burpees, whatever suits you.

+ Get at least seven hours of sleep. This is probably the most difficult part if you are not an easy sleeper or if your head is filled with thoughts or worries. Some ideas include:

  + Sleep in a darkened room.
  + No phone, TV, computer or bright lights one hour before you plan to sleep.
  + Use the 7 x 7 or Rhythm and Blues technique described in Stage 2.
  + Go to bed half an hour earlier than planned.
  + Don't avoid unpleasant thoughts but go into them and notice where in your body you feel them (e.g. the belly or throat). Simply place your hand on that location.[53] You will notice that the thought and related stress will often dissipate on its own. We often get stuck in thoughts and compulsions because we want to avoid them. When I ask you to not think of a red ball for the next minute, you will have a hard time not doing so. The exercise above is an easy way of getting out of the compulsion.

FINAL THOUGHTS

+ Don't attempt things that will fundamentally change your lifestyle in an unsustainable way.
+ Reward yourself for even minor shifts in fibre intake, activity or sleep.
+ It is perfectly fine to go back to a previous stage. This is not a competition, but a way of increasing years of healthy lifetime. Each stage does this!

6. LET'S GET COOKING

'WE SPEND SO MUCH TIME AND MONEY ON DRESSING OUR OUTSIDES. IT'S TIME TO DRESS OUR INSIDES.'

This chapter has two sets of menus. The first one is a quick view of a day and shows you how you can boost your fibre intake by adding foods to your typical intake. The items and fibre-boosting ideas also serve as a guide for when you eat out and want to decide between different dishes. It is really meant to demonstrate that we can easily get to twice the recommended amount of fibre and to three times our current average consumption without much difficulty. So, no excuses!

The second set of menus has the actual recipes for typical foods we all enjoy. They are designed to be simple to make. You don't have to be a Michelin-starred chef to make these, but I guarantee that you will beat all Michelin-starred chefs on the sugar-to-fibre-ratio of your dishes! For those of you who need recipes and practical ideas, I hope the suggested menu items will be enlightening and tasty.

SUPER FIBRE MENU PLAN

I've put together a suggested super-fibre-fuelled menu to give you an idea of what options you have when it comes to planning individual meals. I'm not suggesting you follow this to the letter – it's just a guide – but it gives you an idea of how, by slightly tweaking what you normally enjoy eating, you can easily hit your 30g of fibre a day and more. As I said earlier, fibre is the gift that keeps on giving; the more you have of it the greater the effect.

I have left out any main protein, which you may add to most dishes (e.g. eggs, tofu, meat substitutes, chicken, fish, etc. – most of which have little to no fibre). The suggested ingredients are all readily available and easy to prepare.

In total, this menu delivers close to double the recommended daily amount of fibre and about three to four times what the typical person consumes today. In other words, there is no excuse for not feeding your very fibre-starved dæmon, who in return will gift you with many healthy years of life.

Breakfast (⅓ of your daily need): Muesli consisting of rolled oats, frozen berries, yogurt and chopped walnuts, mixed together. Grate in an apple, some milk for consistency and sprinkle with linseeds. (This will provide around 11g fibre).[54] You can soak the oats overnight in the fridge, and if you use chia seeds instead of the oats the fibre content increases by another 5g, getting you up to half of your daily need.

Snack (⅙ of your daily need): Roasted nuts and 1 passion fruit. (This will provide around 5.5g fibre.)[55]

Lunch (⅓ of your daily need): Grilled vegetable wrap with hummus, beans/falafel in a wholemeal tortilla. (This will provide around 10g fibre.)[56]

Snack (¼ of your daily need): Avocado on oatcakes or multigrain bread sprinkled with lime, coriander and seeds. (This will provide around 8g fibre.)[57]

Dinner (½ of your daily need): Spaghetti with pesto, broccoli and a side of spinach salad with tomato and seeds. (This will provide around 14g fibre.)[58]

Dessert (⅕ of your daily need): High-fibre brownies – raw cacao, wholegrain flour, sweeten with prunes or dates. (This will provide 5-11g of fibre.)[59]

Movie snack (¹⁄₂₀ of your daily need): Popcorn. (This will provide 1.5g of fibre.)[60]

SOME FAVOURITE DISHES

On the following pages, you'll find recipes for some favourite dishes we all enjoy. As you can see, the tweaks are minimal and I have not tried to create dishes with the maximum amount of fibre. All I have done is to take the learnings from the previous chapter and substitute equivalent ingredients. White rice for brown rice, white pasta for wholegrain, and sneak in seeds, pulses or nuts wherever possible. I hope that your takeaway will be that it is really not that big a deal to sneak fibre back into our daily dishes. In a way these strategies take you back to the way our ancestors ate and how some healthy populations on earth still enjoy their food today.

CHILLI TOFU STIR-FRY

Serves 4

Preparation time:
5 minutes, plus
marinating

Cooking time:
12 minutes

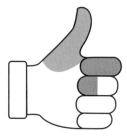

Sugar-to-fibre ratio: 1.4
% daily fibre needs: 22%

A favourite dish the world over with many variations. It originates from east Asia, where the wok is the perfect utensil. The origin of the wok can be traced to the Han dynasty (200BCE) in China but became popular for stir-frying only during the Ming dynasty (14th–17th century).

225g firm tofu, drained and cubed
2 tbsp light soy sauce
2 tbsp sesame oil
2 carrots, cut into matchsticks
175g mangetout, halved
175g small broccoli florets
1 red pepper, seeded and thinly sliced
125g beansprouts
2 tbsp sweet chilli sauce (see box below for how to
*   make this from scratch)*
1 tbsp sesame seeds

SWEET CHILLI SAUCE

1 red chilli, diced
2 pitted prunes, diced
1 tbsp water or olive oil

1. Blend all the ingredients together until they form a smooth paste/sauce.

2. Add additional water or oil until it has the right consistency of a thick-flowing sauce.

1. Place the tofu in a shallow dish with the soy sauce. Cover and set aside to marinate for 10 minutes.

2. Heat the sesame oil in a wok. Add the tofu and stir-fry for 5 minutes. Remove and set aside.

3. Add all the vegetables and stir-fry for 3–4 minutes until just tender. Stir in the tofu.

4. Stir in the sweet chilli sauce and soy sauce from the marinade and cook for 1 minute until heated through.

5. Sprinkle with the sesame seeds and serve immediately.

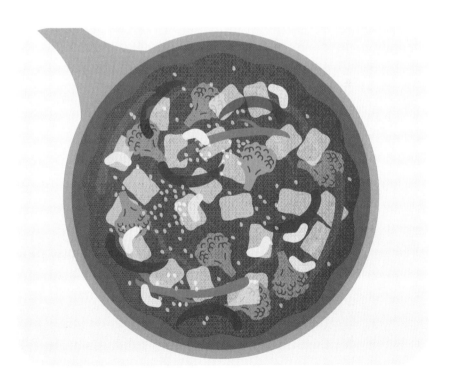

CHICKEN TIKKA MASALA

Serves 4

Preparation time:
45 minutes (includes
making the tikka masala
paste from scratch)

Cooking time:
20 minutes

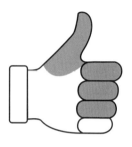

Sugar-to-fibre ratio: 3
% daily fibre needs: 12%

Seen as one of the canonical Indian dishes, but there is much debate as to its origin. Was it created on the Indian subcontinent or by a Pakistani chef in Glasgow to suit the European palate? Either way it has become one of the most desired dishes in Europe and North America.

2 tbsp vegetable oil or ghee
1 onion, thinly sliced
2 garlic cloves, crushed
6 boneless, skinless chicken thighs, cut into strips
2 tbsp tikka masala paste (see box below for how to
*   make this from scratch)*
1 x 400g can chopped tomatoes
450ml hot vegetable stock
*   (1 stock cube in hot water)*
225g natural yogurt
2 tbsp mango chutney
boiled wild or brown rice, to serve

TIKKA MASALA PASTE

½ tsp coriander seeds
½ tsp cumin seeds
½ tsp cayenne pepper
½ tsp smoked paprika
1 tsp garam masala
1 tbsp tomato purée
1 tbsp peanut oil
3 tsp salt
1 small piece of fresh ginger,
*   finely diced*
1 red chilli, chopped

½ tbsp desiccated coconut
1 tbsp almond flour
5 sprigs of fresh coriander,
*   chopped*

1. Lightly fry the dried spices and tomato purée in the oil.

2. Add the salt, ginger, chilli, coconut, almond flour and fresh coriander and grind together or blend in a food processor.

1. Heat the oil or ghee in a large pan. Add the onion and cook over a medium heat for 8 minutes until tender and golden. Add the garlic and chicken and cook, stirring occasionally, for 5 minutes or until golden brown.

2. Stir in the tikka masala paste, then add the tomatoes and hot stock. Bring to the boil, then reduce the heat to low, cover the pan and simmer for 15 minutes or until the chicken is cooked through.

3. Stir in the yogurt and mango chutney and heat through very gently without boiling.

4. Serve hot on a bed of boiled wild or brown rice.

For added fibre, sprinkle with 3 tsp black onion (nigella) seeds.

SPAGHETTI BOLOGNESE

Serves 4

Preparation time:
15 minutes

Cooking time:
40 minutes

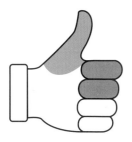

Sugar-to-fibre ratio: 2
% daily fibre needs: 10%

Another fusion recipe. Its origins are obviously in Bologna, Italy (Bolognese ragù), but my Italian friends generally disavow the dish, and it is rarely found outside of tourist areas in Italy. It was probably created by Italian immigrants to the US or UK, who blended the Italian ragù sauce with the popular and easily cooked spaghetti pasta. While we will never know for sure, it is yet another example of what happens when cultures blend for the delight of children and adults alike.

2 tbsp olive oil
1 onion, finely chopped
2 carrots, diced
3 celery sticks, diced
2 garlic cloves, crushed
450g minced beef (or meat substitute)
2 tbsp tomato purée
300ml red wine
1 x 400g can chopped tomatoes
a few sprigs of fresh thyme
450g wholegrain spaghetti
4 tbsp freshly grated Parmesan
sea salt and freshly ground black pepper

1. To make the sauce, heat the oil in a large pan, add the onion, carrots and celery and fry over a medium heat for 10 minutes or until tender. Add the garlic and cook for 1 minute.

2. Add the beef and cook, stirring occasionally, until browned. Stir in the tomato purée and wine and bring to the boil. Add the tomatoes and thyme, and season with salt and pepper. Bring back to the boil, then reduce the heat and simmer gently for 20 minutes.

3. Cook the spaghetti in a large pan of lightly salted boiling water according to the packet instructions. Drain well, then return to the pan.

4. Add the Bolognese sauce and toss together. Divide among four shallow bowls and sprinkle with Parmesan before serving.

For added fibre, sprinkle with crushed roasted walnuts (crush in a mortar and brown in a non-stick pan).

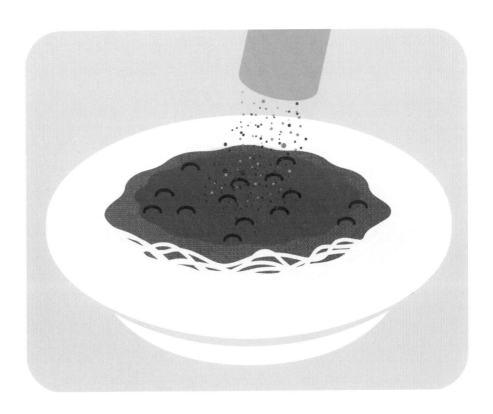

PESTO BEAN BURGER

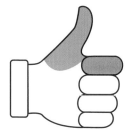

Sugar-to-fibre ratio: 0.8
% daily fibre needs: 31%

Who would have thought that the origins of the burger would be so hotly contested. Did it come from Hamburg, Germany, or did Dutch immigrants to the new world create it? Was it invented multiple times? After all, putting a piece of shredded meat between two slices of bread is not really rocket science and I'm sure the burger has existed in some form or other since the invention of sliced bread.

2 x 400g cans butter beans, rinsed and drained
2 small onions, finely chopped
2 garlic cloves, crushed
2 red chillies, deseeded and diced
2 tbsp red pesto sauce
a few sprigs of fresh coriander
2 medium eggs, beaten
50g grated reduced-fat Cheddar cheese
4 tbsp fat-free fromage frais
plain flour, to dust
spray oil
4 tsp or more of sweet chilli sauce (see page 120)
sea salt and freshly ground black pepper

1. Put the beans in a food processor or blender with the onions, garlic, chillies, pesto, coriander, beaten egg, cheese and fromage frais. Add some seasoning and blitz to a stiff paste. For a rougher texture, you can mash the beans with a potato masher and then stir in the other ingredients. Chill in the fridge until ready to cook.

2. Divide the mixture into four portions and shape each one into a patty with your hands. Dust lightly with flour.

3. Lightly spray a large shallow frying pan with oil and place over a medium heat. When it's really hot,

add the bean burgers and cook for 5 minutes on each side until crisp and golden.

4. Serve immediately with some chilli sauce.

For added fibre, add 1 tbsp guacamole (see page 129).

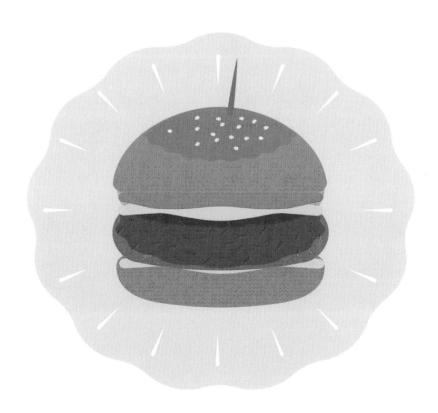

COD WITH LENTILS AND BUTTERNUT SQUASH

Serves 4

Preparation time:
10 minutes

Cooking time:
35 minutes

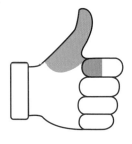

Sugar-to-fibre ratio: 0.6
% daily fibre needs: 80%

Cod, also called the 'British gold', has been an important fish since the Viking times (800CE) and a staple food for most people living around the north Atlantic. It is no wonder that it featured prominently in the Brexit negotiations.

3 tbsp olive oil, plus extra to brush
450g butternut squash, peeled, seeded and diced
2 x 400g cans green lentils, rinsed and drained
4 tsp balsamic vinegar
2 garlic cloves, finely chopped
300g cherry tomatoes
2 red onions, cut into wedges
4 x 150g frozen cod fillets
2 tsp harissa paste
sea salt and freshly ground black pepper
chopped parsley, to serve

1. Preheat the oven to 180°C/350°F/Gas 4.

2. Brush a roasting pan with a little oil, then add the butternut squash. Roast in the oven for 10 minutes.

3. Turn the squash and push it to the edges of the roasting pan. Add the lentils to the centre of the pan. Drizzle with the balsamic vinegar and mix in the garlic and a little salt and pepper.

4. Arrange the cherry tomatoes and red onion around the edge. Put the cod fillets on top of the lentils. Mix together the harissa paste and oil, and drizzle over the fish and vegetables.

5. Roast for 25 minutes or until the fish and squash are cooked. Serve in bowls, sprinkled with parsley.

GUACAMOLE

Serves 4–6

Preparation time:
10 minutes

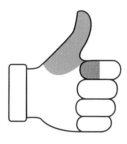

Sugar-to-fibre ratio: 0.4
% daily fibre needs: 31%

Finally, a dish that has a less contested origin: Mexico. Avocados have been cultivated in Central America for at least 10,000 years and their many nutrients, especially fibre, make them a powerhouse of health.

2 ripe avocados, peeled and mashed
2 small tomatoes, chopped
1 red onion, finely chopped
1 garlic clove, finely chopped
juice of 2 limes
2 tbsp chopped fresh coriander
sea salt and freshly ground black pepper

1. In a bowl, mix together the avocados, tomatoes, onion, garlic, lime juice and coriander. Season to taste. Chill in the fridge.

For added fibre, add roasted sunflower seeds.

SWEDISH CHOCOLATE OATBALLS

Makes 35 balls

Preparation time:
20 minutes

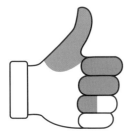

Sugar-to-fibre ratio: 2.7
% daily fibre needs: 11%

A recent addition to the world's culinary delights, this Swedish invention (although some Danes dispute this) most likely made its debut during the Second World War when people were looking for an easy recipe for a sweet snack that did not require wheat, which was rationed at the time.

150g rolled oats
2 tbsp water or cold coffee
1 tsp vanilla sugar or vanilla extract
3 tbsp cocoa powder (unsweetened)
200g dates (pitted and skinned) or date paste
150g butter at room temperature
100g desiccated coconut, ground almonds or sesame
    seeds, to coat

1. Mix all the ingredients, except the coconut, almonds or sesame seeds, together and knead by hand.

2. Take bite-sized amounts and roll into 35 balls.

3. Roll each ball in the coating and put in the fridge to chill before serving.

HOT BERRIES WITH DARK AND WHITE CHOCOLATE

Serves 4

Preparation time:
20 minutes

Cooking time:
15 minutes

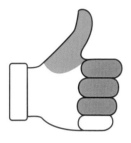

Sugar-to-fibre ratio: 2.9
% daily fibre needs: 10%

And finally, a dish with no origin. Except for the chocolate, which has its origins in central America, where it was used primarily as a drink. 'Chocolate' comes from the Aztec word 'xocóatl', meaning bitter water. The cocoa bean found its way to Europe and almost immediately the 'bitter water' of the Aztecs became less healthy in Europe through the addition of copious amounts of sugar. During the 19th century, the current solid form was created. Many of today's brand names, such as Fry's, Nestlé, Cadbury and Hershey's, were early pioneers in creating the modern chocolate bar. Cocoa is one of the richest sources of fibre.

500g frozen berries (raspberries, blueberries,
   strawberries, blackberries)
100g walnuts or almonds, crushed
100g white chocolate, crushed or grated
100g dark chocolate, crushed or grated

1. Preheat the oven to 180°C/350°F/Gas 4.

2. Place the frozen berries in an ovenproof container. Sprinkle with the crushed walnuts or almonds. Sprinkle with the white and dark chocolate.

3. Place in the oven for 15 minutes, or until the chocolate has melted and slightly caramelised.

7. BEYOND FIBRE

'FIBRE, PHYSICAL ACTIVITY AND FUN ARE THE LONGEVITY TRINITY. YOU CAN SAFELY IGNORE EVERYTHING ELSE.'

By now, I hope I've convinced you that by increasing the amount of fibre in your diet, you can enjoy incredible benefits including a longer, healthier life. I hope you've come to appreciate what an affordable option fibre is for most people – and therefore what a powerful tool it can be for improving the health of humanity as a whole.

THE POWER OF THREE

Despite being a powerful force on its own, it's my belief that fibre works even better as part of a three-way approach: my healthy longevity trinity.

Don't worry, I'm not about to tell you that you have to start meditating for hours a day or take up an extreme exercise regime (although moving more is part of it). Rather, I'm going to explain how lightly modifying two other aspects of your life in line with your fibre intake will create the optimal environment for long-term well-being.

If we take a step back and ask, 'What has been the biggest threat to us humans?' then historically the number one killer has been infectious diseases and continues to be in the developing world with close to 40% of deaths.[61,62]

LOW INCOME COUNTRIES (PER CENT OF DEATHS)

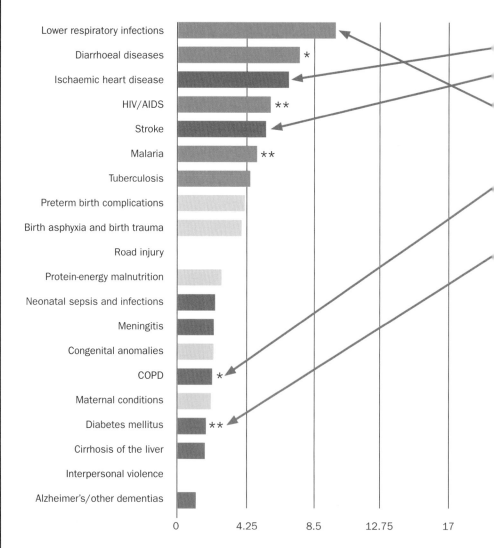

INFECTIOUS DISEASE RELATED
AFFLUENCE/LIFESTYLE/OLD AGE RELATED
DEPRIVATION RELATED
OTHER

Lower respiratory infections	
Diarrhoeal diseases	*
Ischaemic heart disease	
HIV/AIDS	**
Stroke	
Malaria	**
Tuberculosis	
Preterm birth complications	
Birth asphyxia and birth trauma	
Road injury	
Protein-energy malnutrition	
Neonatal sepsis and infections	
Meningitis	
Congenital anomalies	
COPD	*
Maternal conditions	
Diabetes mellitus	**
Cirrhosis of the liver	
Interpersonal violence	
Alzheimer's/other dementias	

0   4.25   8.5   12.75   17

HIGH INCOME COUNTRIES (PER CENT OF DEATHS)

* POTENTIAL IMPACT OF FIBRE
** HIGH IMPACT OF FIBRE AND PHYSICAL ACTIVITY

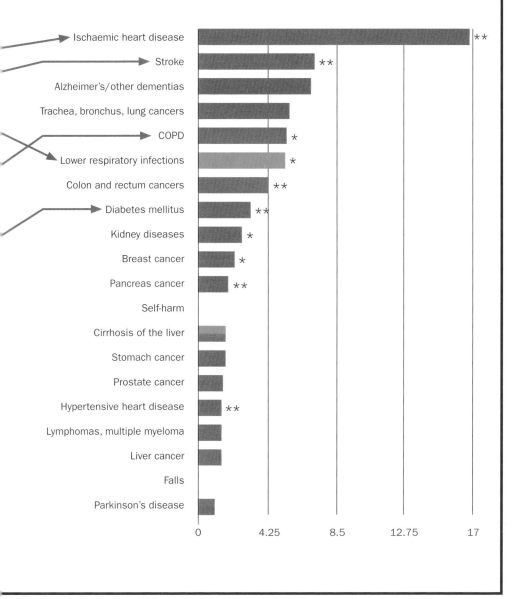

As affluence has grown, a powerful combination of sanitation, vaccination, medical technology and the use of antibiotics has forced the threat to recede. We have basically drained the swamp and – COVID-19 notwithstanding – have continuously reduced infectious diseases as a result.

Technology, medicines and better nutrition have all helped push that historical threat to the fringes and we now live longer. But are we living these longer lives as healthily as possible? It seems not, as our new safer lives have brought the risk of new diseases, many of which are a result of modern lifestyles and habits.

Some of them are obvious, such as smoking; the resultant health issues from which have a significant impact on longevity.[63] But others are more insidious, for example our attitudes to nutrition and physical activity.

How much attention do you think a new drug should get that in the last year alone has been shown to:

+ reduce the risk of death by over 10%
+ reduce the risk of heart attacks and stroke by over 10%
+ reduce the incidence of digestive tract cancers by 10–45%
+ reduce the incidence of breast cancer by over 10% and mortality from breast cancer by over 25%

and has been tested on millions of people, with no side effects, except maybe reducing depression by 24%? See www.fiber4life.com/fiber-facts.

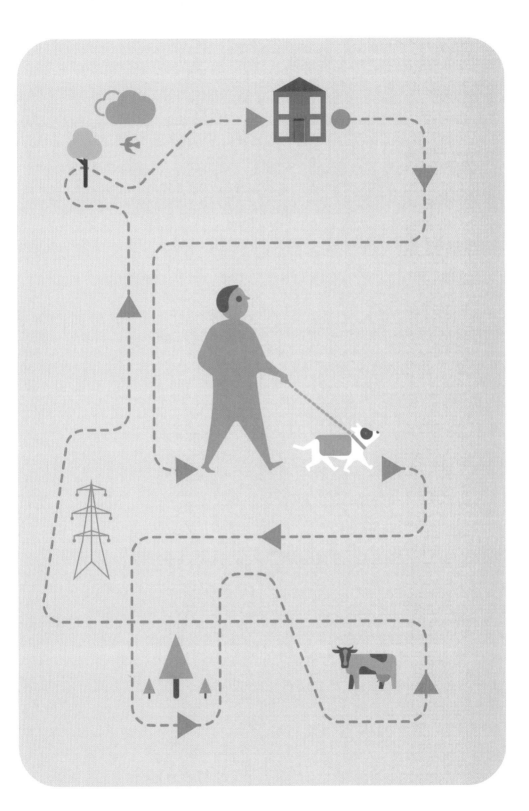

MOVE MORE

Over the previous chapters we have discussed the importance of nutrition and how an increase in our fibre intake can reap many benefits. It's the same story with our approach to physical activity. I'm not talking about a huge change of lifestyle or becoming a super athlete, going to the gym all the time. I've used the term 'physical activity' and not 'exercise' for a reason: moderate additional physical activity can have the same beneficial effects on healthy longevity as fibre.

Being active is one of the most significant things we can do to improve our health. Recent research suggests that sedentary lifestyles could be responsible for 69,000 deaths per year in the UK alone.[64] That's 11% of all deaths, with low physical activity being blamed for an increase in cancer, diabetes and heart disease, and a cost to the NHS of £700 million per year. An earlier, more comprehensive study puts the overall societal costs at over $2.4bn for the UK (and for the world at $64bn; as a comparison, more than half of the countries on earth have a smaller GDP than that).[65]

We may not think we're in the sedentary lifestyle bracket but if we sit down for six hours or more a day – whether at home or at work – then that's exactly where we are.

Roughly, for every hour of physical activity (brisk walking) per week there is >10% reduction of all-cause mortality (a similar effect is seen also for cardiovascular disease and to a lesser level for certain cancers).[66] Imagine that combined with the other health benefits I've discussed throughout this book.

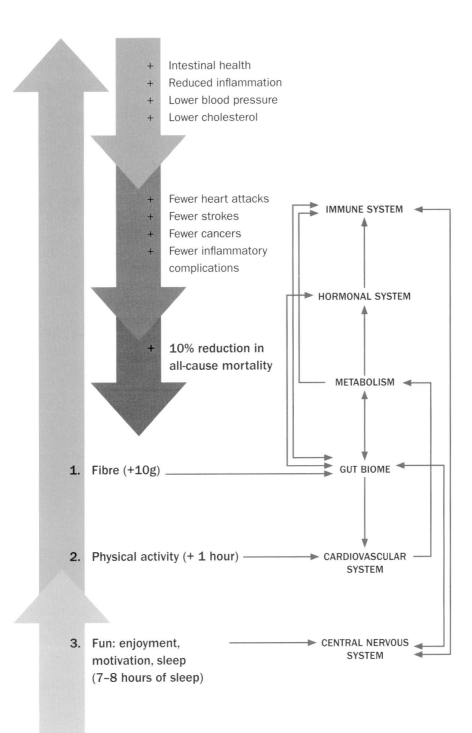

+ Intestinal health
+ Reduced inflammation
+ Lower blood pressure
+ Lower cholesterol

+ Fewer heart attacks
+ Fewer strokes
+ Fewer cancers
+ Fewer inflammatory
  complications

+ **10% reduction in
  all-cause mortality**

IMMUNE SYSTEM

HORMONAL SYSTEM

METABOLISM

1. Fibre (+10g) ——————————————— GUT BIOME

2. Physical activity (+ 1 hour) ——————— CARDIOVASCULAR
                                         SYSTEM

3. Fun: enjoyment,
   motivation, sleep ————————— CENTRAL NERVOUS
   (7–8 hours of sleep)   SYSTEM

In addition, a lot of digestive conditions are improved by increasing physical activity; for example a common prescription for constipation is taking regular walks, a couple of times a day.

It doesn't end there. Moderate additional physical activity has a similar effect on inflammation and our immune system as fibre. This is because they both most likely boost the same beneficial gut microbes and therefore produce the same benefits as discussed in Chapter 4. But how?

Again, the science on this is still in its infancy, but results from a range of studies in animals and humans point to a set of reasonable explanations: physical activity influences the autonomic nervous system which in turn influences the involuntary constriction and relaxation of the muscles of the intestine, causing changes in mucus formation and secretion of fluid into the gut. This in turn alters the environment for the gut bacteria and thus changes the relative abundance of these bacteria. Some of these studies have found that even moderate physical activity has an impact on the type and diversity of our gut flora and when returning to a sedentary lifestyle that the microbiome tends to return to its earlier, less happy state.[67]

As we can see, the benefits of an increased intake of fibre and physical activity are synergistic. These greater-than-the-sum-of-their-parts benefits are particularly pertinent to being healthy later in life, because the more we move now the more lively we will be as we age.

Additionally, physical activity also has a benefit for our cardiovascular system by boosting the strength of our heart, burning excess energy, strengthening our muscles and bones, and a host of positive psychological benefits (improved mood and concentration, reduced pain, better sleep).

FUN: ENJOY YOURSELF AND GET SOME SLEEP

All good things come in threes and there's one more element to add to fibre and physical activity to make up my healthy longevity trinity. While there is some interesting research backing up the presence of a strong correlation for this third principle, the case for a causation is still tenuous. So, I would ask you to consider it as more of a personal belief based on experience rather than hard science. And it can be summed up in one word: enjoyment. That is to say, if we get pleasure out of what we're doing, then we do it more. I'm not saying that enjoying what you do directly ensures you live longer – although this may be true.[68] What I mean is that if you build fibre and physical activity into the things you already enjoy – the meals and the activities – then it'll be a lot easier for you to maintain those life-giving behaviours. And there is an important feedback loop: physical activity and a healthy gut can directly cause more enjoyment.

In order to add fun to your fibre and physical activity formula, one emerging area in scientific research is suggesting we also get sufficient sleep.

Studies using twins show that sleeping 7–8 hours a night is correlated with >20% lower risk of all-cause mortality.[69] When you get a good night's sleep you are not only happier the following day, but it seems you add years to your life. The lack of sufficient sleep is at such a massive scale that the Centers for Disease Control and Prevention estimates that a third of the population is not getting sufficient sleep with dire consequences in terms of heart disease, obesity/type 2 diabetes, inability to cope with stress and depression.

So there you have it. There are three pillars to our story: fibre, physical activity and enjoyment (sleep). Get these right and you can pretty much ignore the snake oil and the latest trend that separates you from your hard-earned money. This is why my Anti-diet plan builds on these insights.

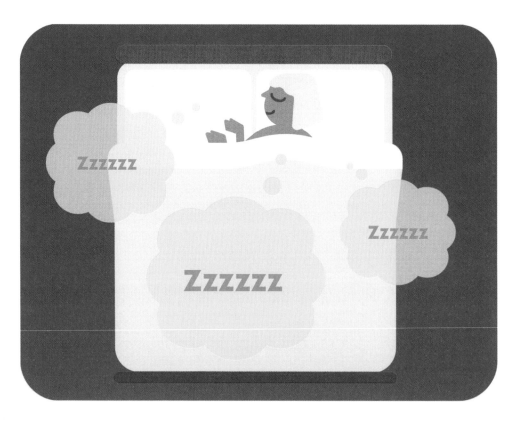

NOW IT IS YOUR TURN

This is not a cookbook, an exercise manual or a self-help book, and I am neither a chef nor a personal trainer nor your shrink. But I can guarantee you this: if you add a handful of raspberries and some seeds to your wholegrain breakfast cereal, and some legumes, nuts and whole grains to your lunch and dinner, you'll be increasing your fibre intake by at least 50%. And if you combine this with an extra 10–15 minutes on your morning walk, you'll be decreasing your all-cause mortality by over 10%. All of this on the back of things you enjoy and a good night's sleep and you will age gracefully like a good wine. My before and after picture is not an overweight person transforming into a cover model, but the grim reaper being told to come back in a decade because there is some livin' and lovin' to be done. Now over to you and let me provoke you a little.

FIBRE

No pain, no gain simply isn't true when you look at the data. With nutrition there's no pain in eating fibre whatsoever; what's high in fibre isn't less tasty. It's no hardship to eat more raspberries, avocados and wholegrain bread is it? Why don't you start today; even better, why don't you smuggle fibre into your loved ones' diet? There is no greater gift you could give. Just smile to yourself, knowing that you are giving them the one thing money can't buy.

PHYSICAL ACTIVITY

Even if you're not a person who enjoys exercise, there are many things you can do to increase the amount you move. Walking is an obvious one, but I'm not talking about power-walking around your locale. Why not become a flâneuse or flâneur (the art of strolling while contemplating life and the world)? Walking can also be a good excuse for some 'me time' (which in itself has a lot of mental health benefits) or a way of catching up with podcasts or the latest audiobook.

If you have a dog then adding another 10 minutes to the daily walk should be no hardship (and the dog loves it) or if you have kids why not find an additional 20 minutes to make them really tired (it pays off with your own sleep later on)?

Love computer games? Then try games that involve physical activity, such as *Beat Saber*, *Sprint Vector* or *BoxVR*. And if your work requires you to sit down, then using a standing desk will ensure that you'll spend part of the day on your feet.

FUN (ENJOYMENT/SLEEP)

Enjoyment is as powerful a tool as increasing fibre and physical activity: it's the glue that binds them together and the reason why you'll do them. It's not about changing your mindset and becoming happy, it's not about mindfulness or anything like that. At a very primitive level, see what it is you enjoy and attach the right nutrition and physical activity to it. It's that simple. Why not list the things you enjoy doing and select the ones that could incorporate food and physical activity? For example, I love cooking and, to the chagrin of my neighbours and wife, I also play loud music and do some embarrassing dance moves while cutting vegetables or stirring the stew. They probably fear that the healthy nutrition and physical activity will prolong their suffering. And the evidence for getting enough sleep is growing day by day. Sleep longer to live longer. My guess, based on data from current research, is that for every additional hour of sleep (up to 8), you gain an additional 5–10 hours of life.

Why not try some of the suggestions for the Anti-Diet Plan from Chapter 5 today and see what parts work for you?

> **FIBRE + PHYSICAL ACTIVITY +FUN = >10 MORE YEARS OF HEALTHY LIFE**

HEALTH BY STEALTH

It seems simple, but the messages the world gives tell you otherwise: you have to change your life, you have to transform yourself. You'd be forgiven for thinking that improving your health is hard and is going to be painful. Well I say that isn't the case! Enjoying the benefits that living well can bring you will make you want to live a better life.

It's health by stealth, no pain all gain.

As a scientist, I can go into great detail about the benefits of increasing our fibre intake on a very deep chemical and biological level. But I've also seen from a personal perspective, helping people shift their nutrition, how it can transform lives and that's what inspires such passion in me about fibre. The more we learn about our microbiome the more we understand how great its impact on our lives is.

Keeping our gut happy and well fed has a huge impact on our health and well-being. There's a wealth of evidence to support that fact – and it's growing fast. By looking after our microbiome we improve the health of our heart and blood circulation, reduce inflammation and strengthen our hormonal and immune systems. It saves healthcare systems billions – and it saves lives.

So my final message to you is this. Forget about cutting out X or restricting Y; forget diets and supplements and the latest snake oil. They are, by and large, money-making machines. Don't listen to those who want to make you feel lacking or scared, it only helps their bank account. Don't waste your time asking government to regulate things, they are generally the last ones to wake up. Take the focus off reducing fat, sugar or carbs. Instead, enjoy the freedom that simply adding more fibre to your diet can bring. Enjoy tasty, satisfying food. Enjoy a little more physical activity and sleep. Enjoy living a longer, happier, healthier life – by simply adding the years you and your loved ones deserve.

Now you know. No excuses!

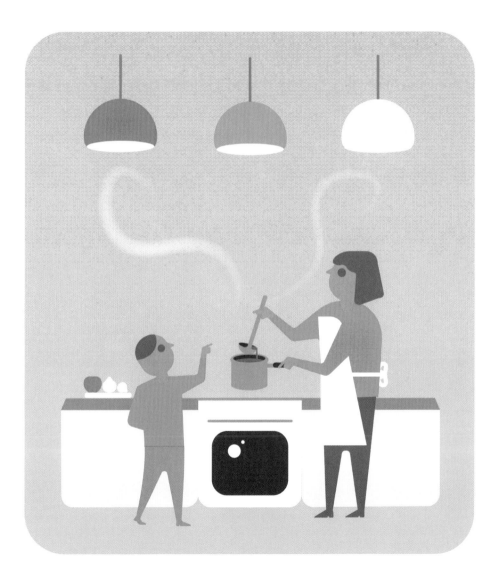

TOP 10 FAQs

1 Why is obesity increasing even though sugar consumption has steadied? The overconsumption of most macronutrients, especially simple carbohydrates, such as sugar (and under-consumption of fibre, with decreasing physical activity) is at such a high level, average body weights will continue to rise. Think of it like a bucket with a hole that will continue filling if the amount of water added (read sugar and over-consumption of other macronutrients) is more than can leave from the hole (read fibre). There may also be a connection to the increased use of antibiotics (not proven). In livestock, use of antibiotics is linked to significant weight gain, presumably by interfering with the gut flora; and the same may be happening in humans, although to what extent this is relevant in terms of societal impact is still unclear.[70] The lower levels of physical activity that most of us, and especially children, experience today compared to even a generation ago further contributes to the increase in obesity.

2 Has the Japanese diet changed over the past century and has that had any detrimental health effects? It indeed has and not for the better. During the 60s over three-quarters of the Japanese diet (in terms of calories consumed) consisted of carbohydrates. (The exact amount of fibre in this number is unknown, but I assume much of it was complex carbs/fibre and thus resulting in a long life expectancy. The low-carb diet people should take a note of this.) Today, the Japanese diet contains less than 60% carbo-hydrates and a larger proportion of it is simple sugars, which also shows up as an increase in dental decay. Japan is currently reaping the benefits of its past diet, but will increasingly catch up with the rest of the industrialised nations if it continues on its current path. Incidentally, in the 60s, the Japanese diet consisted of around 12% fat[71] (as percent of calories consumed) compared to a western diet of close to 40% today. The high-fat diet people should take note of this. I should mention that the Japanese diet is not the best diet imaginable, but it goes far along the path to a healthy diet. Most traditional diets have significant similarities (high fibre, low sugar, whole fresh ingredients). Unfortunately, often traditional diets are abandoned in favour of convenient ones, once populations become more affluent.

3 Does the genetic makeup of a person have an influence on how nutrients are metabolised? It most likely does, but the extent is difficult to assess. Let's not forget that there is a strong evolutionary advantage if a species can extract every last bit of energy from its diet. So it's no surprise that humans with a better ability to do so used to have a better chance of survival during times of famine. With the abundance of food in our times, this advantage has become a liability. This is called the thrifty gene hypothesis and is not proven, however one example is from the Pima Native American tribe, who originally lived in a desert environment with high food scarcity and have among the highest obesity rates when consuming a typical American diet, support this hypothesis. There are over 40 genes identified that may influence our ability to extract energy from food, or impact our satiety/satiation. As usual, how much is nature or nurture will probably come down to the statement: nurture determines how your nature shines through.

4 Are there any supplements that can have a significant positive impact on healthy longevity? In general, unless there is an underlying deficiency, taking supplements is a bad idea. Study after study shows that they either are a waste of money (i.e., do nothing) or can be harmful (because we are effectively overdosing). One exception is Vitamin D where, especially for those living in northern latitudes who may have a deficiency, supplementation has been shown to be beneficial, and potentially vitamin B12 for those on a strictly vegan diet. Of course, there is the placebo effect and if taking something harmless like vitamin C makes you feel better, maybe there is some rationale. I have to admit that whenever I feel a cold coming on I do take an aspirin with vitamin C hoping for some placebo effect.

5 What is the particular importance of the combination of the three elements of healthy longevity: fibre, physical activity and fun (well rested)? These three have the biggest impact on our healthy longevity and, more critically, they are synergistic. Motivation/fun (with sleep constituting the most important element) energises physical activity and gives us a desire to shift our nutrition to healthier alternatives. Healthier nutrition (fibre) makes us feel better in ourselves and enables us to move more and get better rest, primarily via stabilising blood sugar levels.[72] More physical activity encourages better sleep patterns and a higher degree of general motivation. The three elements can be implemented by yourself and do not rely on any other kind of structure or programme.

6 How do I determine if a fact is relevant and can be relied on? Never rely on a single study or fact. For example, 'the reduction of the number of pirates is correlated with an increase in global warming', as the Pastafarians humorously claim. This is a fact, but irrelevant as there is no causation linking the two (to my knowledge). I see this type of statement again and again in the media. This is why looking across multiple sources of evidence or meta analyses have a particular value.

Also, always look at the actual number in conjunction with the percentages. A drug that reduces mortality from a disease by 33% may sound great but the relevance of this drug is fundamentally different if there are 3 people in total that catch that disease every year rather than 3 million. And what if that very same drug causes mortality from another side effect?

Individual anecdotes are another potential minefield. Just because John's grandma is still smoking in her 90s or Gwyneth feels 10 years younger after putting some new serum on her skin, it is in no way evidence for anything. This is where influencers can lead us astray in the echo chambers we populate.

Finally, always be suspicious when reasonableness takes the place of hard evidence. For example, it is reasonable that detoxing may remove bad things from our bodies, but there simply is no proof that it shows a measurable health benefit (beyond fibre + gut bacteria).

In that vein, I hope that you look at all the evidence presented in this book with a healthy degree of scepticism and feel empowered to form your own view based on more sources than just this book.

7 Which sources are reliable for scientific information? In general, it is helpful to read the set of original studies and not rely on what the media is telling you, especially the tabloids who dramatise everything and typically only focus on the latest individual study result (and often get it wrong). When looking at the evidence yourself, it is often sufficient to read the abstract and the results of the study (this is often published online even if the article is not available without a subscription). This can go a long way to form your view without taking many hours of work. Lay publications, such as *Scientific American* and *New*

Scientist are well researched and generally well written. Meta analyses are, in my view, the best sources as they often review the issue and provide a summary of many properly vetted studies. The Cochrane Foundation (www.cochrane.org) and the Cochrane Library are great resources for finding the latest meta analyses on a wide range of topics.

8 What about alternative medicine and holistic approaches? They should be no more or less subject to scrutiny than anything else. They either have a positive (or negative) effect, or not (holistic or otherwise). So far I have not seen any intervention or approach that can even remotely compete with fibre (ideally, in combination with physical activity and fun). The fact that an approach is steeped in history and ancient culture does not make it inherently valuable. For example, bloodletting is probably one of the oldest (at least 2500 years old) medical interventions known to many human cultures (the red and white striped pole in front of barber shops still visible today was a sign that bloodletting was performed at the premises). It was prescribed for pretty much every disease thinkable. Egyptian, Greek, Roman, Jewish, Christian, Islamic, Ayurvedic and traditional Chinese medicine all have practiced it or are still practising it today. How could such a widely practised medicine possibly be wrong? Well, it is provably wrong as it simply does not have the effect claimed, once a proper level of scrutiny is applied. More problematically, it has been one of the main causes of death throughout the ages. One famous example is that of George Washington, who was killed by bloodletting. He had developed a throat infection and the approach used was to drain him, over a period of 9–10 hours, of over half of his blood.[73] Bloodletting started to wane once evidence (and not hearsay or case studies) was collected that showed quite the opposite: not a cure but a death sentence. Remember, it is ultimately not possible to prove anything right, but it is absolutely possible to prove something wrong.

9 What are practical solutions for improving healthy longevity at societal level? Obviously this needs a much broader discussion as it involves learning from past mistakes, extracting insight from successful programmes (these exist and are mostly at micro level), and learning how to mobilise healthcare systems, and informing and energising broad segments of the population. Briefly, my view is that there are two flanking levers that we can implement at societal level that are also economically feasible. There is not enough space here to delve into the details of each idea, so please see this more as a thought starter, rather than a fully worked out framework.

a. Ensure that there are the right incentives for increasing fibre:

i. Low sugar-to-fibre ratio products (e.g., less than 4:1) should have lower VAT type taxes or incentives to make them more affordable for low income households and incentivise manufacturers to incorporate more fibre, and more wholegrain/ food ingredients into their products. For example, it is a travesty that in the UK flapjacks or chocolate chip biscuits are VAT exempt, but many healthier products, such as roasted nuts, are not. The saved medical cost to our healthcare systems from higher fibre consumption more than compensates for the lost taxes/incentives for higher fibre inclusion.[74] Alternatively, a small tax on sugar and sweeteners (as a raw material and not on the final product, in the same way we tax other types of energy), would compensate for a significant subsidy for fibre-containing products. It would also force companies to innovate products that contain less sugar/sweetener and more fibre. Many worry that such a tax on sugar itself will increase food costs and harm low income families disproportionately. What people do not realise is that a higher cost of certain raw madterials will simply shift consumption to alternatives and, as chapter 5 shows, the alternatives are not necessarily more expensive.

ii. School meals must be measured on the level of fibre present in the meal and the level of fibre consumed (i.e., net of waste). While various food pyramids/food group frameworks are used as a guideline, and nutrition standards do tend to favour fruit, vegetable, and grain components, the actual amount of fibre in school meals is still too low[75] and from my discussions with school nutritionists in the USA and the UK, the main concern is the amount of calories, salt, sugar and saturated/trans fat. Again fibre is a 'nice to have', but even the nutritionists have a difficult time telling me how much fibre their kids are eating. While much progress has been made[76], we are still far from the mark and the level of waste on fruit and vegetables is still over 50%. I want to emphasise that school meals play a very important function, especially for low-income families, and there simply is no trade-off between providing a nutritious meal and one that has sufficient levels of fibre to ensure that a child has the best start in life, avoids obesity and grows up the healthiest it can be.

b. Ensure that there is increasing awareness around the powerful benefits of fibre:

i. Establish sugar-to-fibre ratio information on product packaging with a simple-to-understand traffic light logo. While many regulatory bodies are moving forward with similar ideas for the macro-nutrients, they often ignore fibre (for example, the front of the package colour coded information in the EU/UK shows calories, fat and saturated fat, sugar and salt only). If this book is right and fibre powerfully outweighs all other considerations, then it should be the only prominent information on the package. Studies show that consumers are confused by current nutrition information as a basis for making sound decisions. They are simply overwhelmed. So maybe less is more in this case.[77] Also in my own dealings with food regulatory bodies in the UK and EU, the utter lack of understanding of fibre is shocking.

ii. Adjust school science education to reflect the value of fibre and how to incorporate it into one's lifestyle. This should include homework that incorporates parental co-operation to ensure the broader family also grows their knowledge.

iii. Adjust medical school curricula to study the impact of all life-saving medicines versus the preventative impact of higher dietary fibre consumption. The medical establishment's awareness of fibre is more of an afterthought and nutrition science is currently inadequately taught at most medical schools.[78] The adjusted curriculum should include all medical doctors, dentists, nurses and nutritionists.

iv. Make it far more costly for manufacturers to have false or redundant nutrition claims including a false depictions of sugar (e.g., coconut blossom nectar) and fibre (e.g., there are ingredient suppliers who sell certain products as fibre but a simple taste test tells you that it contains simple sugars). As fibre will increasingly step into the limelight this issue will continue to grow.

10 Where do you see the future developments in the fibre space? In terms of the science, we are truly at the beginning of our understanding of how our gut and various fibres interact and the myriad effects on our body systems. My best guess is that the impact of fibre on inflammation will play an increasingly central role as inflammation causes all kinds of problems across most body systems. We discussed in chapter 4 some of the more speculative areas and I would think that the long-term impact on our brain will increasingly come to the fore.

In terms of societal attention and financial investment, I believe we stand before a mega trend. Just see how protein has captured the language of our times (high protein this, super protein that). The main reason, in my opinion, is that it was associated with beautiful bodies (e.g., initially body builders followed by other athletes) and popular diets (e.g., Atkins). Fibre has much more going for it. The science on the healthfulness of fibre is incredibly solid and expanding by the minute. Policy makers will soon wake up to the fact that, if they want their societies to be healthier and more productive, ignoring fibre any longer is knowingly wasting resources and human potential.

ENDNOTES

1   Farvid, M. S., Spence, N. D., Holmes, M. D., and Barnett, J. B. (2020) 'Fibre consumption and breast cancer incidence: A systematic review and meta analysis of prospective studies', *Cancer*, 126 (13), 3061–75.

2   For a review of the replication problem, see: Baker, M. (2016) '1,500 scientists lift the lid on reproducibility', *Nature*, 533 (7604), 452–454.

3   Yang, Y., Zhao, L. G., Wu, Q. J., Ma X., Xiang Y. B. (2015) 'Association between dietary fibre and lower risk of all-cause mortality: a meta-analysis of cohort studies', *Am J Epidemiol*, 181 (2): 83–91.

4   Circa 37,000 road accident-related deaths p.a.; see https://www.worldatlas.com/articles/how-many-people-are-killed-in-road-accidents-in-the-us.html; All cause number of deaths (2.8million), see https://www.cdc.gov/nchs/fastats/deaths.html

5   Vaughan, A., Frazer, Z. A., Hansbro, P. M., and Yang, I. A. (2019), 'COPD and the gut-lung axis: the therapeutic potential of fibre', *Journal of Thoracic Disease*, 11 (Suppl 17), S2173–80.

6   Fibre, through its central influence on our gut microbiota, is known to have a positive effect on inflammation in general, and diseases of the airways that involve an immune response from the body in particular. Among many other benefits of fibre, it is metabolised by some of our gut bacteria into short-chain fatty acids. These have a profound effect on our immune system in terms of reducing inflammation and promoting a wide range of other benefits. Several studies also show that the positive effects relate to the development of protective immunity and reduced immune system-linked tissue damage when lungs are infected with the flu or COVID-19. See: Maslowski, K. M. et al. (2009) 'Regulation of inflammatory responses by gut microbiota and chemoattractant receptor GPR43', *Nature*, 461: 1282–1286.

Trompette, A. et al. (2014) 'Gut microbiota metabolism of dietary fibre influences allergic airway disease and hematopoiesis', *Nat. Med.*; 20: 159–166.

Corrêa-Oliveira, R. et al. (2016) 'Regulation of immune cell function by short-chain fatty acids', *Clin Transl Immunology*, 5 (4), e73.

Ríos-Covián, David et al. 'Intestinal Short Chain Fatty Acids and their Link with Diet and Human Health', *Frontiers in Microbiology*, 7, 185.

Trompette, A. et al. (2018) 'Dietary Fibre Confers Protection against Flu by Shaping Ly6c− Patrolling Monocyte Hematopoiesis and CD8+ T Cell Metabolism', *Immunity*, 48 (5), 992–1005.e8.

Tirawattanawanich, C. (2001) 'The Modulating Effects of Dietary Fibre and Short-Chain Fatty Acids on Enterocyte Differentiation, Maturation, and Turkey Coronavirus Infection', Dissertation submitted to the Faculty of Virginia Polytechnic Institute & State University.

Hughes, Christine et al. (2011) 'Galactooligosaccharide supplementation reduces stress-induced gastrointestinal dysfunction and days of cold or flu: a randomized, double-blind, controlled trial in healthy university students.' *The American Journal of Clinical Nutrition*, 93 (6), 1305–1311.

The broad effect extends to other diseases of the lungs such as COPD: Kan, Haidong et al. (2008) 'Dietary fibre, lung function, and chronic obstructive pulmonary disease in the atherosclerosis risk in communities study', *American Journal of Epidemiology* vol. 167, 5. While all deliberate infection studies have been done in animals, one study with over 400 students showed a 40% reduction in the percentage of days with cold or flu in normal-weight individuals with 5g of additional fibre consumption per day.

7   Modelling of shifts in current diets shows that a mild shift can have a greater than 15% reduction in greenhouse gas emissions. See: Horgan, Graham W. et al. (2016) 'Achieving dietary recommendations and reducing greenhouse gas emissions: modeling diets to minimise the change from current intakes', *The International Journal of Behavioral Nutrition and Physical Activity*, 13, 46.

8   For the same amount of protein, grains emit 95% less greenhouse gases than beef, and nuts emit 95% less than chicken. See: Poore, J., & Nemecek, T. (2018) 'Reducing food's environmental impacts through producers and consumers', *Science*, 360 (6392), 987–992. For a good visualisation see ourworldindata.org.

9   The current debates range between seeing the following culprits: 1. fat due to its high energy content (or fat in combination with sugar); 2. the protein leverage hypothesis, which suggests that protein consumption is prioritised over other macronutrients (i.e., we eat until we get enough protein independent of the overall calorie consumption); 3. sugar as the driver of artificial starvation (explained in the book), carbohydrates in general as the ultimate sources of sugar. None have to my knowledge seriously looked at the lack of fibre or more importantly to the sugar-to-fibre ratio. There are other hypotheses; for example, an increasing use of antibiotics has been proposed as one possible candidate. It is well-known that antibiotics used in animal feed lead to rapid weight gain due to their impact on the gut microbiome and studies in humans support this too. See: Turta, O., & Rautava, S. (2016) 'Antibiotics, obesity and the link to microbes – what are we doing to our children?', *BMC Medicine*, 14, 57. https://doi.org/10.1186/s12916-016-0605-7

10   World Health Organization, Global and regional food consumption patterns and trends.

11   Based on USA Food and Drug Administration definition of daily values for consumption of macronutrients and calories. In developed countries a total of 3,440kcal/capita are consumed (53% from carbohydrates, 12% from protein, 34% from fats), against a target of 2000kcal/capita. National Institute

of Health, USA, and see also National Academy of Sciences, Engineering, and Medicine: www.nap.edu; https://ods.od.nih.gov/Health_Information/Dietary_ Reference_Intakes.aspx; http://who.int/nutrition/ topics/3_foodconsumption/en/. See Table 50, https:// www.ers.usda.gov/data-products/sugar-and-sweeteners-yearbook-tables/sugar-and-sweeteners-yearbook-tables/#U.S. Consumption of Caloric Sweeteners https://www.nal.usda.gov/sites/default/files/fnic_ uploads//macronutrients.pdf#:~:text=Dietary%20 Reference%20Intakes%3A%20Macronutrients%20 Nutrient%20Function%20Life%20Stage,increases%20 absorption%20of%20fat%20soluble%20vitamins%20 and%20precursors

12 Top end of range, see: Reynolds A. et al. (2019) 'Carbohydrate quality and human health: a series of systematic reviews and meta-analyses', *The Lancet* 393, (10170), 434–445. For lower end of range: Micha, R. et al. (2014) 'Global, regional, and national consumption levels of dietary fats and oils in 1990 and 2010: a systematic analysis including 266 country-specific nutrition surveys', *BMJ*, 348: g2272.

13 Public Health England, Food and Nutrition Board, Institute of Medicine, National Academies, https://www. ncbi.nlm.nih.gov/books/NBK56068/table/ summarytables t4/?report=objectonly.

14 For maximum levels, see: Bilsborough, S., Mann, N. (2006) 'A review of issues of dietary protein intake in humans', *Int J Sport Nutr Exerc Metab.*, 16 (2): 129–52. For a review of deleterious impact see: Delimaris, I. (2013) 'Adverse Effects Associated with Protein Intake above the Recommended Dietary Allowance for Adults', *ISRN Nutr.* 126929. Levine. M.E., et al. (2014) 'Low Protein Intake Is Associated with a Major Reduction in IGF-1, Cancer, and Overall Mortality in the 65 and Younger but Not Older Population', *Cell Metabolism*, 19 (3), 407–417.

15 There is of course also the correlation between overall energy consumption and obesity, but this analysis shows the way to tackle the problem. Often people assume that reducing one of the nutrients – for example, the more energy dense component, namely fat – is the quickest way, but this analysis suggests increasing fibre.

16 The analysis was conducted using available data on macronutrient consumption for comparable nations (similar GDP/capita, advanced healthcare system, similar levels of education). For sugar there is no reliable total sugar consumption available that is measured in a similar way across regions. Thus the lower number of added sugar was used (the real number will be 20–50% higher and will polarise the existing numbers even further as there is reason to believe that the Japanese (followed by the Italians and the USA) also consume less sugar-containing natural products in the diet due to the propensity of vegetables and pulses in the diet. A sensitivity analysis was also made to ensure that differences in smoking prevalence and exercise do not change the conclusion. The total difference does not exceed a difference of four months of longevity. The following sources were used to assemble the data:

Macronutrient consumption: Zhang, R., Wang, Z., Fei, Y., Zhou, B., Zheng, S., Wang, L., Huang, L., Jiang, S., Liu, Z., Jiang, J., and Yu, Y. (2015) 'The Difference in Nutrient Intakes between Chinese and Mediterranean, Japanese and American Diets', *Nutrients*, 7 (6), 4661–88.

Sugar consumption: USDA and Statista (https://www. statista.com/outlook/40100000/141/confectionery/ italy)

Health expenditure and financing: OECD (Organisation for Economic Co-operation and Development) Statistics on health expenditure and financing. In order to compare like-for-like, the raw numbers were adjusted for factor costs (e.g., costs for salaries and medicines are close to 2 x higher in the US, which is unrelated to higher disease burden and should therefore be adjusted). For a discussion see: https://www.cnbc.com/2018/03/22/ the-real-reason-medical-care-costs-so-much-more-in-the-us.html

Obesity-related costs: Harvard University, https://www. hsph.harvard.edu/obesity-prevention-source/ snapshot-of-obesity-related-costs/; Cawley, J., Meyerhoefer, C., (2012) 'The medical care costs of obesity: an instrumental variables approach', *J Health Econ.* 31 (1), 219–30.

Hoque, M. E., Mannan, M., Long, K. Z., Al Mamun, A. (2016) 'Economic burden of underweight and overweight among adults in the Asia-Pacific region: a systematic review', *Trop Med Int Healt,* 21 (4), 458–69.

17 Office for National Statistics, UK. For an interactive map, see: https://www.thesun.co.uk/news/5747126/ how-long-will-you-interactive-map-life-expectancy/

18 In a US study, people with less than $25,000 annual income consumed c. 16% less dietary fibre than people with more than $75,000 annual income. While there are many contributing factors other than diet (accidents, smoking, other diseases, stress, education etc.), a significant correlation can be seen with obesity and related diseases that are positively influenced by higher fibre consumption. See: Storey, Maureen and Anderson, Patricia (2014) 'Income and race/ethnicity influence dietary fibre intake and vegetable consumption', *Nutrition Research,* 34 (10), 844–850; National Health and Nutrition.

Chetty, R., Stepner, M., Abraham, S., et al. (2016) 'The Association Between Income and Life Expectancy in the United States, 2001–2014', *JAMA*, 315 (16), 1750–1766.

Wang, S. Y., Tan, A. S. L., Claggett, B., Chandra, A., Khatana, S. A. M., Lutsey, P. L., Kucharska-Newton, A., Koton, S., Solomon, S. D., Kawachi, I. (2019) 'Longitudinal Associations Between Income Changes and Incident Cardiovascular Disease: The Atherosclerosis Risk in Communities Study', JAMA Cardiol, 4 (12): 1203–1212.

Theodora Psaltopoulou, George Hatzis, Nikolas Papageorgiou, Emmanuel Androulakis, Alexandros Briasoulis, Dimitris Tousoulis (2017) 'Socioeconomic status and risk factors for cardiovascular disease: Impact of dietary mediators', Hellenic Journal of Cardiology, 58 (1), 32–42.

19 Drewnowski, A., Darmon, N. 'Does social class predict diet quality?', Am J Clin Nutr., 2008, 87, 1107-1117. See also: N. Darmon, A. Drewnowski (2015) 'Contribution of food prices and diet cost to socioeconomic disparities in diet quality and health: a systematic review and analysis', Nutrition Reviews, 73 (10), 643–660.

20 Anderson, J. W., Konz, E. C., Frederich, R. C., and Wood, C. L. (2001) 'Long-term weight-loss maintenance: a meta-analysis of US studies', The American Journal of Clinical Nutrition, 74 (5), 579–84.
Headland, M., Clifton, P. M., Carter, S., and Keogh, J. B. (2016) 'Weight-loss outcomes: a systematic review and meta-analysis of intermittent energy restriction trials lasting a minimum of 6 months', Nutrients, 8 (6), 354.
Long, G., et al. (2020) 'Comparison of dietary macronutrient patterns of 14 popular named dietary programmes for weight and cardiovascular risk factor reduction in adults: systematic review and network meta-analysis of randomised trials', BMJ, 369, 696. The success rates are similar even for medical interventions in the case of diabetes: Diabetes Prevention Program Research Group (2009) '10-year follow-up of diabetes incidence and weight loss in the Diabetes Prevention Program Outcomes Study', The Lancet, 374 (9702), 1677–86. [Published correction appears in The Lancet (2009) 374 (9707), 2054.]

21 For a good overview see: Dulloo, A. G., and Montani, J. P. (2015) 'Pathways from dieting to weight regain, to obesity and to the metabolic syndrome: an overview', Obesity Reviews, 16 (Suppl 1), 1–6.

22 Anastasiou, C. A., Karfopoulou, E., and Yannakoulia, M. (2015) 'Weight regaining: from statistics and behaviors to physiology and metabolism', Metabolism, 64 (11), 1395–407.

23 There is also increasing evidence that metabolism adjustments and the resilience of our gut bacteria may play a significant role. For a recent review, see: Fragiadakis, G. K., Wastyk, H. C., Robinson, J. L., Sonnenburg, E. D., Sonnenburg, J. L., and Gardner, C. D. (2020) 'Long-term dietary intervention reveals resilience of the gut microbiota despite changes in diet and weight', The American Journal of Clinical Nutrition, 111 (6), 1127–36.

24 There is some evidence that individuals who engage in active weight maintenance do manage to keep the pounds off, beyond the initial weight loss, and that for most diets a minority of people do manage to achieve meaningful longer-term weight reduction (c. 10–20%). See: Mansoor, N., Vinknes, K. J., Veierød, M. B., and Retterstøl, K. (2016) 'Effects of low-carbohydrate diets v. low-fat diets on body weight and cardiovascular risk factors: a meta-analysis of randomised controlled trials', British Journal of Nutrition, 115 (3), 466–79.

25 Different diets (e.g. carbohydrate reduction versus fat reduction) also appear to have a trade-off between reduction of weight and increase of LDL cholesterol. Ibid.

26 Cunnane, S., Nugent, S., Roy, M., et al. (2011) 'Brain fuel metabolism, aging, and Alzheimer's disease', Nutrition, 27 (1): 3–20.

27 Daly, M. E., Vale, C., Walker, M., Littlefield, A., Albert, K. G., Mathers, J. C. (1998) 'Acute effects on insulin sensitivity and diurnal metabolic profiles of a high-sucrose compared with a high-starch diet', Am J Clin Nutr., 67 (6): 1186–96.

28 It appears that satiation (feeling of being full after a meal) is strongly influenced by food volume and satiety (length of time one feels full) is strongly influenced by the amount of certain macro nutrients, especially protein and fibre. See, Holt SH et al. (1995) 'A satiety index of common foods', Eur J Clin Nutr, 49 (9): 675–90. Bell, E. A. et al. (1998) 'Energy density of foods affects energy intake in normal-weight women', Am J Clin Nutr., 67 (3): 412–20.

29 Public Health England (September 2019) 'Sugar reduction: Report on progress between 2015 and 2018'.

30 Various sugar taxes on beverages have been applied in many countries and regions (e.g., Mexico, France, USA, Finland, Ireland, Hungary). The results all show a reduction in consumption of sugar-sweetened beverages, see, for example: Sánchez-Romero Luz M. et al. (2020) 'Association between tax on sugar sweetened beverages and soft drink consumption in adults in Mexico: open cohort longitudinal analysis of Health Workers Cohort Study', BMJ, 369.

31 To put the impact of insulin in somewhat simplified terms: sugar (glucose) causes an increase in insulin, which in turn leads to higher levels of fat being deposited and, when the insulin crashes, an artificial starvation effect is created (low sugar), which causes us to grab for the next sugar hit. Sugar (fructose) is also metabolised in our liver and plays a role (together with saturated fat and trans fats) in the formation of plaques in our arteries.

32 For a summary of current research see: Fowler, S. P. (2016) 'Low-calorie sweetener use and energy balance: results from experimental studies in animals, and large-scale prospective studies in humans', Physiol Behav., 9384 (16) 30184–6.

33 For a recent review see, Harpaz, D. et al. (2018) 'Measuring Artificial Sweeteners Toxicity Using a Bioluminescent Bacterial Panel', Molecules, 23 (10), 2454. See also a review by Scientific American: https://www.scientificamerican.com/article/artificial-sweeteners-may-change-our-gut-bacteria-in-dangerous-ways/

34 There is no comprehensive study comparing different sweeteners. The hypothesis is that there are no differences between high potency sweeteners (e.g., sucralose, aspartame, aceK, stevia, saccharin) as they are all used in minuscule amounts due to their high levels of sweetness (100–500 x sugar). Presumably, their impact likely comes from the gut-brain interaction. The impact from sugar alcohols (e.g., erythritol, xylitol, sorbitol, maltitol) may be different and have more of a direct effect on the gut flora, as most are consumed in larger amounts as their sweetness is similar or lower than sugar (sucrose).

35 Sweeteners negatively impact the gut flora, may

decrease satiety, alter glucose homeostasis, and are associated with increased caloric consumption and weight gain. See: Pearlman, M., Obert, J., Casey, L. (2017) 'The Association Between Artificial Sweeteners and Obesity', *Curr Gastroenterol Rep.*, 19 (12): 64. Also see Meghan, B., Azad M.B., et al. (2017), 'Nonnutritive sweeteners and cardio-metabolic health: a systematic review and meta-analysis of randomized controlled trials and prospective cohort studies', *Canadian Medical Association Journal*, 189 (28). For research on the impact of sweeteners on the gut microbiome, see: Bian, X., et al. (2017), 'The artificial sweetener acesulfame potassium affects the gut microbiome and body weight gain in CD-1 mice', *PLoS One*, 8, 12 (6).

36 Even in the field of gut health, much of the focus is on pro-biotics and post-biotics, because you can patent the organisms (and prescribe them on a daily basis) and while there seems to be some short-term benefit, it pales in the face of what fibre can deliver free of charge.

37 For a recent overview of where the evidence is the strongest based on multiple meta-analyses, see: Veronese, N., Solmi, M., Caruso, M. G., Giannelli, G., Osella, A. R., Evangelou, E., Maggi, S., Fontana, L., Stubbs, B. and Tzoulaki, I. (2018), 'Dietary fibre and health outcomes: an umbrella review of systematic reviews and meta-analyses', *The American Journal of Clinical Nutrition*, 107 (3), 436–44.

38 One of the markers of ageing is the length of the chromosome caps (called teleomeres). As we age these caps get shorter which result in a number of ageing-related symptoms. Fibre has a high likelihood of a profound impact on reducing the shortening of these teleomeres. See for example: Tucker, L. A. (2018) 'Dietary Fibre and Telomere Length in 5674 U.S. Adults: An NHANES Study of Biological Aging', *Nutrients*, 10 (4): 400.

39 Reynolds, A., Mann, J., Cummings, J., Winter, N., Mete, E., and Te Morenga, L. (2019), 'Carbohydrate quality and human health: a series of systematic reviews and meta-analyses', *The Lancet*, 393 (10170), 434–45.

40 Fibre binds between four and eleven times its weight in water. See: Robertson, J. A. et al. (2000) 'Hydration Properties of Dietary Fibre and Resistant Starch: a European Collaborative Study', *LWT – Food Science and Technology*, 33 (2), 72–79.

41 There is roughly the same number of bacterial cells as there are human cells in our body.

42 Helander, H. F., Fändriks, L. (2014), 'Surface area of the digestive tract-revisited', *Scandinavian Journal of Gastroenterology*, 49 (6), 681–9.

43 Coppa, G. V., Zampini, L., Galeazzi, T., and Gabrielli, O. (2006), 'Prebiotics in human milk: a review', *Digestive and Liver Disease*, 38 (Suppl 2), S291–4.

44 Khan, W. I., and Ghia, J. E. (2010) 'Gut hormones: emerging role in immune activation and inflammation', *Clinical and Experimental Immunology*, 161 (1), 19–27.

45 Smits, S. A., Leach, J., Sonnenburg, E. D., Gonzalez, C. G., Lichtman, J. S., Reid, G., Knight, R., Manjurano, A., Changalucha, J., Elias, J. E. and Dominguez-Bello, M. G.

(2017) 'Seasonal cycling in the gut microbiome of the Hadza hunter-gatherers of Tanzania', *Science*, 357 (6353), 802–6.

46 Not only are healthier foods affordable, but they also satisfy reduced greenhouse gas emissions. For a recent review, see: Reynolds, C. J., Horgan, G. W., Whybrow, S., and Macdiarmid, J. I. (2019) 'Healthy and sustainable diets that meet greenhouse gas emission reduction targets and are affordable for different income groups in the UK', *Public Health Nutrition*, 22 (8), 1503–17.

47 There is a significant correlation between insufficient sleep and obesity (cause is yet unknown). For example, see: Patel, S. R., Malhotra, A., White, D. P., Gottlieb, D. J., and Hu, F. B. (2006) 'Association between reduced sleep and weight gain in women', *American Journal of Epidemiology*, 164 (10), 947–54.

48 Wasalathanthri, S., Hettiarachchi, P., and Prathapan, S. (2014), 'Sweet taste sensitivity in pre-diabetics, diabetics and normoglycemic controls: A comparative cross sectional study', *BMC Endocrine Disorders*, 14 (1), 67.

49 There are fibre supplements that you can also use. In general I would avoid these, but if you find it easier, then pick a few and make your own blend. Remember that fibre binds a lot of water and you should never eat the fibre supplement powder straight, but always dissolve it in lots of water (there is a risk otherwise of choking or obstructing your throat).

50 For every hour of additional moderate physical activity, there is a 10% reduction in mortality.

51 This method quickly tends to put a person into a very relaxed state, where the heartrate variability becomes more regular. It is the same state as one finds in meditation. With practice, you can increase your count to 10.

52 This method anchors the brain to a certain rhythm and, by slowing down the rhythm, it relaxes the mind, helping the person to more easily enter a sleep stage.

53 Briefly, the reason this works is that when avoiding certain thoughts we focus on avoiding them and thus they keep their power over us. When we let the thought happen and notice where in our bodies we feel the thought and 'get in touch with it', our subconscious has a chance to work on it and our attention is naturally brought to ourselves rather than the external irritant. For more on this see: Schellenbaum, P. (1999) *Nimm deine Couch und geh!: Heilung mit Spontanritualen* (Dt. Taschenbuch Verlag).

54 50g rolled oats, 5g fibre/30g chia seeds, 10g fibre; 25g raspberries, 2g fibre; 25g walnuts, 2g fibre; 8g linseed, 2g fibre.

55 30g almonds, 3.5g fibre; 1 passion fruit, 2g fibre.

56 100g falafel/beans and hummus, 7g fibre; tortilla wrap, 2g fibre; 30g grilled vegetable (e.g. peppers), 1g fibre.

57 1 portion/slice of oatcake/bread, 2g fibre; half an avocado, 3.5g fibre; 10g seeds, 2.5g fibre.

58 150g pasta, 7g fibre; 60g pesto, 1g fibre;

3 broccoli spears, 3g fibre; 50g spinach, 1g fibre; 1 small 90g tomato, 1g fibre; 9g sesame seeds, 1g fibre.

59   For one brownie, 8.5g of whole grain flour, 1g fibre; 50g dates or prunes, 4g fibre; 34g unsweetened baking chocolate, 6g fibre.

60   10g portion, 1.5g fibre.

61   Malaria, tuberculosis, leprosy, influenza, smallpox, the plague. The Black Death alone killed close to one third of the population at its height during the mid-fourteenth century and empires such as the Aztec were annihilated by smallpox. See: Byrne, J. P. [ed.] (2008) *Encyclopedia of Pestilence, Pandemics and Plagues* (Greenwood Press).

62   World Health Organization (2016) 'Global disease burden and mortality estimates', 1900–1940 tables ranked in National Office of Vital Statistics, December 1947, Centers for Disease Control and Prevention.

63   The estimates on economic impact from smoking have a wide range. For a comprehensive source that attempts to include all costs (not necessarily borne by taxpayers), see: tobaccoatlas.org.

64   Heron, L., O'Neill, C., McAneney, H., Kee, F., and Tully, M. A. (2019) 'Direct healthcare costs of sedentary behaviour in the UK', *Journal of Epidemiology and Community Health*, 73 (7), 625–9.

65   Ding, D., Lawson, K. D., Kolbe-Alexander, T. L., Finkelstein, E. A., Katzmarzyk, P. T., Van Mechelen, W., Pratt, M. and Lancet Physical Activity Series 2 Executive Committee (2016) 'The economic burden of physical inactivity: A global analysis of major non-communicable diseases', *The Lancet*, 388 (10051), 1311–24.

66   Kraus, W. E., Powell, K. E., Haskell, W. L., Janz, K. F., Campbell, W. W., Jakicic, J. M., Troiano, R. P., Sprow, K., Torres, A., Piercy, K. L. and 2018 Physical Activity Guidelines Advisory Committee (2019) 'Physical activity, all-cause and cardiovascular mortality, and cardiovascular disease', *Medicine & Science in Sports & Exercise*, 51 (6), 1270–81.

67   Allen, J. M., Mailing, L. J., Niemiro, G. M., Moore, R., Cook, M. D., White, B. A., Holscher, H. D. and Woods, J. A. (2018) 'Exercise alters gut microbiota composition and function in lean and obese humans', *Medicine & Science in Sports & Exercise*, 50 (4), 747–57.

Bressa, C., Bailén-Andrino, M., Pérez-Santiago, J., González-Soltero, R., Pérez, M., Montalvo-Lominchar, M. G., Maté-Muñoz, J. L., Domínguez, R., Moreno, D. and Larrosa, M. (2017) 'Differences in gut microbiota profile between women with active lifestyle and sedentary women', *PLoS One*, 12 (2), e0171352.

68   There is some evidence that people who are in the lowest quartile of optimism vs. the highest quartile had a hazard ratio of 0.71 (i.e. 29% reduction) for all-cause mortality. Adding health behaviours, health conditions and depression attenuated but did not eliminate the associations (hazard ratio = 0.91 (9% reduction). It appears, though, that the correlation is more linked to the level of pessimism than the extent of optimism in a person. See: Kim, E. S., Hagan, K. A., Grodstein, F., DeMeo, D. L., De Vivo, I., and Kubzansky, L. D. (2017) 'Optimism and cause-specific mortality: A prospective cohort study', *American Journal of Epidemiology*, 185 (1), 21–9.

Whitfield, J. B., Zhu, G., Landers, J. G., and Martin, N. G. (2020) 'Pessimism is associated with greater all-cause and cardiovascular mortality, but optimism is not protective', *Scientific Reports*, 10 (1), 12609.

69   Hublin, C., Partinen, M., Koskenvuo, M., and Kaprio, J. (2007) 'Sleep and mortality: A population-based 22-year follow-up study', *Sleep*, 30 (10), 1245–53.

70   Stark, C. M., Susi, A., Emerick, J., et al. (2019) 'Antibiotic and acid-suppression medications during early childhood are associated with obesity', *Gut*, 68: 62–69.

71   Matsushita, Yumi et al. (2004) 'Trends in Childhood Obesity in Japan over the Last 25 Years from the National Nutrition Survey', *Obesity Research*, 12: 205–14.

72   Gangwisch, James E. et al. (2020) 'High glycemic index and glycemic load diets as risk factors for insomnia: analyses from the Women's Health Initiative', *The American Journal of Clinical Nutrition*, 111/2: 429–439.

73   Vadakan, Vibul V. (2004) 'The asphyxiating and exsanguinating death of president George Washington', *The Permanente Journal*, 8/2: 76–79.

74   The back of the envelope calculation is simple: Adding 10g of additional fibre to our diet translates to having circa one meal with higher amounts of fibre. The incentives for such a meal would be 30% to make it more attractive (i.e., savings of GBP 1–2, $1.5–3 for the consumer). The savings on obesity alone would pay for at least a third of the additional cost (see chapter 1, The Wealth of Nations) not to mention non-obesity related medical costs (circa 5x higher than the obesity-related costs) and the economic impact of work days lost (on average across developed countries there are about 4–10 days lost per person per year, see: Integrated Benefits Institute publications and Office of National Statistics, www.ons.gov.uk).

75   Bardin, S., Washburn, L., Gearan, E., (2020) 'Disparities in the Healthfulness of School Food Environments and the Nutritional Quality of School Lunches', *Nutrients,* 12(8). The Food Foundation (July 2017) 'UK and Global Malnutrition: The New Normal'.

76   Harvard School of Public Health (March 2014), 'New school meal standards significantly increase fruit, vegetable consumption'.

77   Miller, L. M. S., Cassady, D. L., Beckett, L. A., Applegate, E. A., Wilson, M. D., Gibson, T. N. et al. (2015) 'Misunderstanding of Front-Of-Package Nutrition Information on US Food Products', *PLoS ONE,* 10 (4): e0125306.

78   Womersley, K., Ripullone, K. (2017) 'Medical schools should be prioritising nutrition and lifestyle education', *BMJ* 359; and Macaninch, E., Buckner, L., Amin, P., et al. (2020), 'Time for nutrition in medical education', *BMJ Nutrition, Prevention & Health,* bmjnph-2019-000049.

INDEX

ACKNOWLEDGEMENTS

This book has been a true collaboration. Over the past years many friends, colleagues, people who have listened to my talks and my family have asked the same question, 'Why, if fibre is so important, don't you write a book about it?' I am thankful to all those who asked this question and did not give up on me.

While writing this book, first and foremost my editors Sophie Allen, Wesley Doyle and Hannah Ebelthite, have been a source of inspiration, creative writing and practical advice.

My colleagues at Zendegii and Frill: Mats Lindstrand, Peter Freedman, Anna Hällöv, Jan Åström, Andrew McKinlay, Malin Elinder, Stina and Erik Eriksson, Simon Adolphson, Jonas Stiernström, Jahanshah and Jahansooz Jomehri, Johannes Falk, Erik Nerpin, Duncan Emery, Fatemeh Farahani, Daniel Kohn, Helge Jordan, Hendrik Sabert, Iain McLaughlin, Arun Nagwaney and Katharine Kent, have helped forge the ideas over the years and over numerous challenging discussions into a coherent whole.

Imran Amed gave me the first platform to share the ideas with a broader audience in the fashion and arts world.

Peter Schellenbaum gave me the impetus to look deeper into what is real and find my own vantage point.

My friends Professor Carlo Pozzi, who knows everything about plants; Clara Lombardo, who cooks the best food I have ever eaten; Professor Andrew MacMillan, who is one of the best scientists I have ever worked with; Jean-Yves Ortholand, my go-to-chemistry genius; Todd and Trish Morgan, the best listeners an author could hope for; Bodi Rongen, whose paintings are second to none; and Professor Mikael Elinder, who has the most refreshing view on economics – all have helped ferment my ideas.

My daughters, Noura, Aria and Mina, have proven to be amazing critics and proofreaders, not only of this book, but of everything I do, so that I can grow with them. My nephews, Ali and Amir, have been better than brothers to me (and my sisters-in-law Sedi, Leila and Parinaz) and always willing to try my various concoctions. My sister Shirin always manages to gently shift my perspective for the better and with it my ability to hopefully get my points across. My wife Cecilia has, as ever, kept me focused on what is important, with her journalistic instincts and generosity of spirit.

I also thank you, dear reader, that you are willing to overlook my shortcomings and take some seed from this book that may be of use once it falls on the fertile ground of your mind and is nurtured by your pleasure of trying something new.